Table of Contents

Secret Key #1 - Time is Your Greatest Enemy

Pace Yourself

Wear a watch. At the beginning of the test, check the time (or start a chronometer on your watch to count the minutes), and check the time after every few questions to make sure you are "on schedule."

If you are forced to speed up, do it efficiently. Usually one or more answer choices can be eliminated without too much difficulty. Above all, don't panic. Don't speed up and just begin guessing at random choices. By pacing yourself, and continually monitoring your progress against your watch, you will always know exactly how far ahead or behind you are with your available time. If you find that you are one minute behind on the test, don't skip one question without spending any time on it, just to catch back up. Take 15 fewer seconds on the next four questions, and after four questions you'll have caught back up. Once you catch back up, you can continue working each problem at your normal pace.

Furthermore, don't dwell on the problems that you were rushed on. If a problem was taking up too much time and you made a hurried guess, it must be difficult. The difficult questions are the ones you are most likely to miss anyway, so it isn't a big loss. It is better to end with more time than you need than to run out of time.

Lastly, sometimes it is beneficial to slow down if you are constantly getting ahead of time. You are always more likely to catch a careless mistake by working more slowly than quickly, and among very high-scoring test takers (those who are likely to have lots of time left over), careless errors affect the score more than mastery of material.

Secret Key #2 - Guessing is not Guesswork

You probably know that guessing is a good idea - unlike other standardized tests, there is no penalty for getting a wrong answer. Even if you have no idea about a question, you still have a 20-25% chance of getting it right.

Most test takers do not understand the impact that proper guessing can have on their score. Unless you score extremely high, guessing will significantly contribute to your final score.

Monkeys Take the Test

What most test takers don't realize is that to insure that 20-25% chance, you have to guess randomly. If you put 20 monkeys in a room to take this test, assuming they answered once per question and behaved themselves, on average they would get 20-25% of the questions correct. Put 20 test takers in the room, and the average will be much lower among guessed questions. Why?

1. The test writers intentionally write deceptive answer choices that "look" right. A test taker has no idea about a question, so picks the "best looking" answer, which is often wrong. The monkey has no idea what looks good and what doesn't, so will consistently be lucky about 20-25% of the time.
2. Test takers will eliminate answer choices from the guessing pool

- 5 -

based on a hunch or intuition. Simple but correct answers often get excluded, leaving a 0% chance of being correct. The monkey has no clue, and often gets lucky with the best choice.

This is why the process of elimination endorsed by most test courses is flawed and detrimental to your performance- test takers don't guess, they make an ignorant stab in the dark that is usually worse than random.

$5 Challenge

Let me introduce one of the most valuable ideas of this course- the $5 challenge:

You only mark your "best guess" if you are willing to bet $5 on it.
You only eliminate choices from guessing if you are willing to bet $5 on it.

Why $5? Five dollars is an amount of money that is small yet not insignificant, and can really add up fast (20 questions could cost you $100). Likewise, each answer choice on one question of the test will have a small impact on your overall score, but it can really add up to a lot of points in the end.

The process of elimination IS valuable. The following shows your chance of guessing it right:

If you eliminate wrong answer choices until only this many remain:	Chance of getting it correct:
1	100%
2	50%
3	33%

However, if you accidentally eliminate the right answer or go on a hunch for an incorrect answer, your chances drop dramatically: to 0%. By guessing among all the answer choices, you are GUARANTEED to have a shot at the right answer.

That's why the $5 test is so valuable- if you give up the advantage and safety of a pure guess, it had better be worth the risk.

What we still haven't covered is how to be sure that whatever guess you make is truly random. Here's the easiest way:

Always pick the first answer choice among those remaining.

Such a technique means that you have decided, **before you see a single test question**, exactly how you are going to guess- and since the order of choices tells you nothing about which one is correct, this guessing technique is perfectly random.

This section is not meant to scare you away from making educated guesses or eliminating choices- you just need to define when a choice is worth eliminating. The $5 test, along with a pre-defined random guessing strategy, is the best way to make sure you reap all of the benefits of guessing.

Secret Key #3 - Practice Smarter, Not Harder

Many test takers delay the test preparation process because they dread the awful amounts of practice time they think necessary to succeed on the test. We have refined an effective method that will take you only a fraction of the time.

There are a number of "obstacles" in your way to succeed. Among these are answering questions, finishing in time, and mastering test-taking strategies. All must be executed on the day of the test at peak performance, or your score will suffer. The test is a mental marathon that has a large impact on your future.

Just like a marathon runner, it is important to work your way up to the full challenge. So first you just worry about questions, and then time, and finally strategy:

Success Strategy

1. Find a good source for practice tests.
2. If you are willing to make a larger time investment, consider using more than one study guide- often the different approaches of multiple authors will help you "get" difficult concepts.
3. Take a practice test with no time constraints, with all study helps "open book." Take your time with questions and focus on applying strategies.
4. Take a practice test with time constraints, with all guides "open book."
5. Take a final practice test with no open material and time limits

If you have time to take more practice tests, just repeat step 5. By gradually exposing yourself to the full rigors of the test environment, you will condition your mind to the stress of test day and maximize your success.

Secret Key #4 - Prepare, Don't Procrastinate

Let me state an obvious fact: if you take the test three times, you will get three different scores. This is due to the way you feel on test day, the level of preparedness you have, and, despite the test writers' claims to the contrary, some tests WILL be easier for you than others.

Since your future depends so much on your score, you should maximize your chances of success. In order to maximize the likelihood of success, you've got to prepare in advance. This means taking practice tests and spending time learning the information and test taking strategies you will need to succeed.

Never take the test as a "practice" test, expecting that you can just take it again if you need to. Feel free to take sample tests on your own, but when you go to take the official test, be prepared, be focused, and do your best the first time!

Secret Key #5 - Test Yourself

Everyone knows that time is money. There is no need to spend too much of your time or too little of your time preparing for the test. You should only spend as much of your precious time preparing as is necessary for you to get the score you need.

Once you have taken a practice test under real conditions of time constraints, then you will know if you are ready for the test or not.

If you have scored extremely high the first time that you take the practice test, then there is not much point in spending countless hours studying. You are already there.

Benchmark your abilities by retaking practice tests and seeing how much you have improved. Once you score high enough to guarantee success, then you are ready.

If you have scored well below where you need, then knuckle down and begin studying in earnest. Check your improvement regularly through the use of practice tests under real conditions. Above all, don't worry, panic, or give up. The key is perseverance!

Then, when you go to take the test, remain confident and remember how well you did on the practice tests. If you can score high enough on a practice test, then you can do the same on the real thing.

General Strategies

The most important thing you can do is to ignore your fears and jump into the test immediately- do not be overwhelmed by any strange-sounding terms. You have to jump into the test like jumping into a pool- all at once is the easiest way.

Make Predictions

As you read and understand the question, try to guess what the answer will be. Remember that several of the answer choices are wrong, and once you begin reading them, your mind will immediately become cluttered with answer choices designed to throw you off. Your mind is typically the most focused immediately after you have read the question and digested its contents. If you can, try to

predict what the correct answer will be. You may be surprised at what you can predict.

Quickly scan the choices and see if your prediction is in the listed answer choices. If it is, then you can be quite confident that you have the right answer. It still won't hurt to check the other answer choices, but most of the time, you've got it!

Answer the Question

It may seem obvious to only pick answer choices that answer the question, but the test writers can create some excellent answer choices that are wrong. Don't pick an answer just because it sounds right, or you believe it to be true. It MUST answer the question. Once you've made your selection, always go back and check it against the question and make sure that you didn't misread the question, and the answer choice does answer the question posed.

Benchmark

After you read the first answer choice, decide if you think it sounds correct or not. If it doesn't, move on to the next answer choice. If it does, mentally mark that answer choice. This doesn't mean that you've definitely selected it as your answer choice, it just means that it's the best you've seen thus far. Go ahead and read the next choice. If the next choice is worse than the one you've already selected, keep going to the next answer choice. If the next choice is better than the choice you've already selected, mentally mark the new answer choice as your best guess.

The first answer choice that you select becomes your standard. Every other answer choice must be benchmarked against that standard. That choice is correct until proven otherwise by another answer choice beating it out. Once you've decided that no other answer choice seems as good, do one final check to ensure that your answer choice answers the question posed.

Valid Information

Don't discount any of the information provided in the question. Every piece of information may be necessary to determine the correct answer. None of the information in the question is there to throw you off (while the answer choices will certainly have information to throw you off). If two seemingly unrelated topics are discussed, don't ignore either. You can be confident there is a relationship, or it wouldn't be included in the question, and you are probably going to have to determine what is that relationship to find the answer.

Avoid "Fact Traps"

Don't get distracted by a choice that is factually true. Your search is for the answer that answers the question. Stay focused and don't fall for an answer that is true but incorrect. Always go back to the question and make sure you're choosing an answer that actually answers the question and is not just a true statement. An answer can be factually correct, but it MUST answer the question asked. Additionally, two answers can both be seemingly correct, so be sure to read all of the answer choices, and make sure that you get the one that BEST answers the question.

Milk the Question

Some of the questions may throw you completely off. They might deal with a subject you have not been exposed to, or one that you haven't reviewed in years. While your lack of knowledge about the subject will be a hindrance, the question itself can give you many clues that will help you find the correct answer. Read the question carefully and look for clues. Watch particularly for adjectives and

nouns describing difficult terms or words that you don't recognize. Regardless of if you completely understand a word or not, replacing it with a synonym either provided or one you more familiar with may help you to understand what the questions are asking. Rather than wracking your mind about specific detailed information concerning a difficult term or word, try to use mental substitutes that are easier to understand.

The Trap of Familiarity

Don't just choose a word because you recognize it. On difficult questions, you may not recognize a number of words in the answer choices. The test writers don't put "make-believe" words on the test; so don't think that just because you only recognize all the words in one answer choice means that answer choice must be correct. If you only recognize words in one answer choice, then focus on that one. Is it correct? Try your best to determine if it is correct. If it is, that is great, but if it doesn't, eliminate it. Each word and answer choice you eliminate increases your chances of getting the question correct, even if you then have to guess among the unfamiliar choices.

Eliminate Answers

Eliminate choices as soon as you realize they are wrong. But be careful! Make sure you consider all of the possible answer choices. Just because one appears right, doesn't mean that the next one won't be even better! The test writers will usually put more than one good answer choice for every question, so read all of them. Don't worry if you are stuck between two that seem right. By getting down to just two remaining possible choices, your odds are now 50/50. Rather than wasting too much time, play the odds. You are guessing, but guessing wisely, because you've been able to knock out some of the answer choices that you know are wrong. If you are eliminating choices and realize that the last answer choice you are left with is also obviously wrong, don't panic. Start over and consider each choice again. There may easily be something that you missed the first time and will realize on the second pass.

Tough Questions

If you are stumped on a problem or it appears too hard or too difficult, don't waste time. Move on! Remember though, if you can quickly check for obviously incorrect answer choices, your chances of guessing correctly are greatly improved. Before you completely give up, at least try to knock out a couple of possible answers. Eliminate what you can and then guess at the remaining answer choices before moving on.

Brainstorm

If you get stuck on a difficult question, spend a few seconds quickly brainstorming. Run through the complete list of possible answer choices. Look at each choice and ask yourself, "Could this answer the question satisfactorily?" Go through each answer choice and consider it independently of the other. By systematically going through all possibilities, you may find something that you would otherwise overlook. Remember that when you get stuck, it's important to try to keep moving.

Read Carefully

Understand the problem. Read the question and answer choices carefully. Don't miss the question because you misread the terms. You have plenty of time to read each question thoroughly and make sure you understand what is being asked. Yet a happy medium must be attained, so don't waste too much time. You must read carefully, but efficiently.

Face Value

When in doubt, use common sense. Always accept the situation in the problem at face value. Don't read too much into it. These problems will not require you to make huge leaps of logic. The test writers aren't trying to throw you off with a cheap trick. If you have to go beyond creativity and make a leap of logic in order to have an answer choice answer the question, then you should look at the other answer choices. Don't overcomplicate the problem by creating theoretical relationships or explanations that will warp time or space. These are normal problems rooted in reality. It's just that the applicable relationship or explanation may not be readily apparent and you have to figure things out. Use your common sense to interpret anything that isn't clear.

Prefixes

If you're having trouble with a word in the question or answer choices, try dissecting it. Take advantage of every clue that the word might include. Prefixes and suffixes can be a huge help. Usually they allow you to determine a basic meaning. Pre- means before, post- means after, pro - is positive, de- is negative. From these prefixes and suffixes, you can get an idea of the general meaning of the word and try to put it into context. Beware though of any traps. Just because con is the opposite of pro, doesn't necessarily mean congress is the opposite of progress!

Hedge Phrases

Watch out for critical "hedge" phrases, such as likely, may, can, will often, sometimes, often, almost, mostly, usually, generally, rarely, sometimes. Question writers insert these hedge phrases to cover every possibility. Often an answer choice will be wrong simply because it leaves no room for exception. Avoid answer choices that have definitive words like "exactly," and "always".

Switchback Words

Stay alert for "switchbacks". These are the words and phrases frequently used to alert you to shifts in thought. The most common switchback word is "but". Others include although, however, nevertheless, on the other hand, even though, while, in spite of, despite, regardless of.

New Information

Correct answer choices will rarely have completely new information included. Answer choices typically are straightforward reflections of the material asked about and will directly relate to the question. If a new piece of information is included in an answer choice that doesn't even seem to relate to the topic being asked about, then that answer choice is likely incorrect. All of the information needed to answer the question is usually provided for you, and so you should not have to make guesses that are unsupported or choose answer choices that require unknown information that cannot be reasoned on its own.

Time Management

On technical questions, don't get lost on the technical terms. Don't spend too much time on any one question. If you don't know what a term means, then since you don't have a dictionary, odds are you aren't going to get much further. You should immediately recognize terms as whether or not you know them. If you don't, work with the other clues that you have, the other answer choices and terms provided, but don't waste too much time trying to figure out a difficult term.

Contextual Clues

Look for contextual clues. An answer can be right but not correct. The contextual clues will help you find the answer that is most right and is correct. Understand the context in which a phrase or statement is made. This will help you make important distinctions.

Don't Panic

Panicking will not answer any questions for you. Therefore, it isn't helpful. When you first see the question, if your mind goes blank, take a deep breath. Force yourself to mechanically go through the steps of solving the problem and using the strategies you've learned.

Pace Yourself

Don't get clock fever. It's easy to be overwhelmed when you're looking at a page full of questions, your mind is full of random thoughts and feeling confused, and the clock is ticking down faster than you would like. Calm down and maintain the pace that you have set for yourself. As long as you are on track by monitoring your pace, you are guaranteed to have enough time for yourself. When you get to the last few minutes of the test, it may seem like you won't have enough time left, but if you only have as many questions as you should have left at that point, then you're right on track!

Answer Selection

The best way to pick an answer choice is to eliminate all of those that are wrong, until only one is left and confirm that is the correct answer. Sometimes though, an answer choice may immediately look right. Be careful! Take a second to make sure that the other choices are not equally obvious. Don't make a hasty mistake. There are only two times that you should stop before checking other answers. First is when you are positive that the answer choice you have selected is correct. Second is when time is almost out and you have to make a quick guess!

Check Your Work

Since you will probably not know every term listed and the answer to every question, it is important that you get credit for the ones that you do know. Don't miss any questions through careless mistakes. If at all possible, try to take a second to look back over your answer selection and make sure you've selected the correct answer choice and haven't made a costly careless mistake (such as marking an answer choice that you didn't mean to mark). This quick double check should more than pay for itself in caught mistakes for the time it costs.

Beware of Directly Quoted Answers

Sometimes an answer choice will repeat word for word a portion of the question or reference section. However, beware of such exact duplication – it may be a trap! More than likely, the correct choice will paraphrase or summarize a point, rather than being exactly the same wording.

Slang

Scientific sounding answers are better than slang ones. An answer choice that begins "To compare the outcomes…" is much more likely to be correct than one that begins "Because some people insisted…"

Extreme Statements

Avoid wild answers that throw out highly controversial ideas that are proclaimed as established fact. An answer choice that states the "process should used in certain situations, if…" is much more likely to be correct than one that states the "process should be discontinued completely." The first is a calm rational statement and doesn't even make a definitive, uncompromising stance, using a hedge word "if" to provide wiggle room, whereas the second choice is a radical idea and far more extreme.

Answer Choice Families

When you have two or more answer choices that are direct opposites or parallels, one of them is usually the correct answer. For instance, if one answer choice states "x increases" and another answer choice states "x decreases" or "y increases," then those two or three answer choices are very similar in construction and fall into the same family of answer choices. A family of answer choices is when two or three answer choices are very similar in construction, and yet often have a directly opposite meaning. Usually the correct answer choice will be in that family of answer choices. The "odd man out" or answer choice that doesn't seem to fit the parallel construction of the other answer choices is more likely to be incorrect.

Top 20 Test Taking Tips

1. Carefully follow all the test registration procedures
2. Know the test directions, duration, topics, question types, how many questions
3. Setup a flexible study schedule at least 3-4 weeks before test day
4. Study during the time of day you are most alert, relaxed, and stress free
5. Maximize your learning style; visual learner use visual study aids, auditory learner use auditory study aids
6. Focus on your weakest knowledge base
7. Find a study partner to review with and help clarify questions
8. Practice, practice, practice
9. Get a good night's sleep; don't try to cram the night before the test
10. Eat a well balanced meal
11. Know the exact physical location of the testing site; drive the route to the site prior to test day
12. Bring a set of ear plugs; the testing center could be noisy
13. Wear comfortable, loose fitting, layered clothing to the testing center; prepare for it to be either cold or hot during the test
14. Bring at least 2 current forms of ID to the testing center
15. Arrive to the test early; be prepared to wait and be patient
16. Eliminate the obviously wrong answer choices, then guess the first remaining choice
17. Pace yourself; don't rush, but keep working and move on if you get stuck
18. Maintain a positive attitude even if the test is going poorly
19. Keep your first answer unless you are positive it is wrong
20. Check your work, don't make a careless mistake

Case Management Concepts

Case Management/Case managers

Case management is a collaborative and trans-disciplinary practice. It assesses the client's total situation and addresses the needs and problems found in that assessment. It is a means for improving client health, wellness and autonomy. Case Managers act within their profession and the boundaries of their competence, based on their education, skills, moral character, licensing and credentials, and experience. They recognize that everyone has the right to be treated with dignity and self-worth in obtaining quality services and cost-effective interventions and outcomes.

Case Managers provide advocacy, communication, and education, identify service resources, and facilitate services. Case Managers recognize that case management is guided by the principles of autonomy, beneficence, nonmaleficence and justice. Case management/managers strive to have the individual reach an optimum of wellness and functional capability benefiting the support systems, healthcare delivery systems, and the various reimbursement systems. Possession of a CCM credential does not indicate any specific level of capability beyond the achievement of certification. The Health Centers Consolidation Act incorporated case management into its definition of required primary health services.

Client assessment

The initial assessment must be a comprehensive and thorough attempt to develop an accurate profile of the client and the client's problem. The initial assessment may be done on an intake assessment form containing pre-established questions or may be construction of a written narrative of their social history. In either case, it will cover the background of the current problem, current condition, living arrangements, relationships, and work experience. Part of the assessment must include the reason the client is seeking help as well as the initial or presenting problem.

Discussion of the problem leads to what the client requires to bring stability and resolution. The client's personal strengths (e.g. education) and environment (family support) should be documented. Assessment of the client's ability to reason and understand options is a part of the assessment. The assessment is the foundation for the development of an individual plan for service or treatment.

Individualized treatment plan

An individualized plan takes into account the support and resources within the client's family, friends and community. The plan takes advantage of the client's resources in addressing the outstanding or immediate problems. The plan addresses all of the issues raised in the patient's assessment. The plan should include incremental steps toward improvement as well as expected outcomes. Use of formal agencies (e.g. mental health, Easter Seals) as well as folk support/community organizations (church grief support group, ESL tutoring, social organizations) available to assist with a particular issue are important to include in the plan. Development of good individualized plans requires the Case Manager have knowledge of and a relationship with people and places that welcome your clients and provide the experiences or support they need.

Case monitoring

Continued planning and monitoring takes into account changes in the client's health, living circumstances, and the success or failure of the links/transfer/referrals in the treatment plan. It is the Case Manager's responsibility to monitor the services provided to your client. You need to be certain the treatment or services you authorized is being provided or used. All referrals should send reports at specified intervals. Referrals to informal (folk) support groups may need you to contact them or require your professional assessment to determine the success or failure of the services provided, as the group may not have the resources to provide you with the information. Progress toward the goals in the individualized plan may need modifications or revisions, or notations that goals were met. Reassessing the client allows adjustment of the timeline created in the initial assessment and restructuring of services needed. It provides the material needed to prepare a report on the success of case management, including all savings achieved.

Written patient records

Written patients records provides the following:
- Records the actions, and the reason for those actions, taken by Case Managers
- Provides the basis for reporting the costs and savings due to use of case management
- Allows others to manage the case in the absence of the assigned manager
- Provides history and perspective for long and complex cases
- Is necessary in the case of legal action to provide suitability of the care

Remember that all conversations and information about a case fall within the patient-provider privilege and must follow disclosure rules.

Domains of case management

The knowledge domains are as follows:
- Processes and relationships encompass interpersonal relationships including communication and interviewing, case documentation, clinical problem-solving, and negotiation and conflict resolution
- Healthcare management covers medical case management including aspects of acute and chronic illness and disability and the cost saving goals/objectives of case management, healthcare ethics, legal aspects of case management and clinical pharmacology
- Community resources and support requires knowledge of the various levels of care, community resources and support programs, rehabilitation services, and public benefit programs
- Service delivery includes managed care and cost containment procedures, strategies and cost benefit analysis, healthcare benefits and delivery system, wellness concepts and strategies, case management models, and healthcare and disability-related legislation
- Psychosocial intervention includes family dynamics, multicultural and neuropsychological assessment, mental health concepts, substance use/abuse/addiction, managed behavioral healthcare, and psychosocial aspects of chronic illness and disability

- Rehabilitation case management includes disability compensation systems, job analysis/modification/accommodation, vocational assessment, job development and placement, ergonomics, and life-care planning

Managing a patient's care

The eight steps of managing a patient's care are:

1) Case finding happens through referrals: diagnosis-driven, high-dollar referrals or repeated service requests
2) Assessment phase begins with the information that triggered the referral, contacting the patient if further action is warranted, obtaining signed consent forms, and establishing client rapport
3) Planning includes contacting the patient's healthcare providers to obtain treatment plans, then developing the individualized plan
4) Reporting includes desired outcomes, progress toward the outcomes, cost of care with and without case management and savings due to case management
5) Obtaining approval requires documentation signed by the client (or their guardian)
6) Coordination means acting as liaison, coordinator and communicator with everyone who is interested or plays a part in the case of the patient
7) Follow-up/monitoring is a key component of the Case Manager's job. Ensuring that all providers and referrals send reports and updates is vital to maintaining the patient's records and preparing evaluations
8) Evaluation is a dynamic function

The overall strategies and goals must be revised and evaluated after every patient contact and progress report.

SMART goal setting

SMART is an acronym for remembering how to set goals. Every goal must be analyzed to ensure it meets the SMART criteria.

- Specific goals state a number, date, task, etc. to be accomplished. There is no doubt or confusion as to what constitutes achievement of the goal
- Measurable goals mean the action can be measured to see if achievement has occurred
- Achievable takes into account the starting point and all extenuating circumstances
- Realistic goals are a function of measurable and achievable
- Timely sets the goal at an appropriate time in the overall picture of the case

Patient's advocate

In the role of the patient's advocate, the Case Manager is held to a "reasonable standard of care." This requires knowledge of what the standard of care is for the condition. This knowledge is obtained through education and up-to-date information on trends in medical, surgical and rehabilitation therapeutics. It is important the Case Manager understand the appropriateness of the procedure/provider to the patient's case. The Case Manager is not only responsible for their own actions in managing a case, but also the relationship between the patient and any vendors she recommends. Incidents that occur and are reported by either the vendor or the patient, must be investigated with the findings documented and an action plan detailed.

Initial assessment categories

The eight categories covered in the initial assessment meeting with the client are:

1) Cognitive function must be assessed to determine if the client can speak for themselves or if they need a proxy present to answer questions or participate in decision making
2) Diagnosis/medical conditions must be captured and a determination made of areas that may require the Case Manager's intervention
3) Medications are an area where the Case Manager can detect potential problems with drug administration or interactions and arrange assistance if financial barriers exist
4) Care access involves evaluation of services for coordination of the services, obtaining providers or transportation and negotiating costs
5) Functional status covers activities of daily living (ADL), instrumental activities of daily living (IADLs), and fall prevention
6) Social situation evaluates the patient's support system and arranges social work intervention if needed
7) Nutritional status impacts the overall health of the patient and the effectiveness of medication
8) Emotional status is the recognition of depression and other emotional disorders that can negatively impact the well-being of the patient, care plan and desired outcomes

Functional status of patient

Three areas of determining the functional status of a patient are the following:

- Activities of Daily Living (ADL) include basic functions such as the ability to dress, bathe, feed and toilet oneself

The level of independence is based in part on environmental factors: are stairs involved, is equipment needed to provide mobility, etc.

Instrumental Activities of Daily Living (IADLs) include the ability to do housework, shop, and prepare meals.

Barriers in any of these areas may affect the ability to heal effectively or obtain/prepare food. Fall prevention looks at the history of the patient as well as their future.

Case Managers "tell and sell" their role

Case Management referrals come from a variety of sources: flagged by dollar caps on services or the diagnosis (ICD-9 or CPT) code, number of admissions over a period of time, or assigned due to the type of insurance carrier covering the event (e.g. Worker's Comp).

If a Case Manager approaches their role as a reporter gathering information then provides analysis of the information, they will be perceived as contributors to the care plan as opposed to simple observers without pertinent input/contributions. The Case Manager must tell about the patient then sell the concept of case management of the individualized treatment plan.

Disease management vs. case management

Case management oversees an individual patient, whereas disease management focuses on groups of patients with diagnostic conditions that historically have high financial costs and will benefit from integrated and systematic management of treatment. The goal of disease management is to reach individuals at the earliest possible time in the disease cycle.

Assessment of the patient in relation to the disease's risks allows planning and intervention services at appropriate times to reduce both the chronic nature of the disease and the cost complications. The following diseases have demonstrated the effectiveness of disease management: diabetes, asthma, cardiovascular disease, multiple sclerosis, and arthritis to name a few. Only thorough patient interviews will it be determined if an individual needs disease management.

MSE process

Case Manager's use observation in order to document a client's mental status, the client's situation, actions, speech and appearance are taken into account in an abbreviated assessment (e.g. eminent hospitalization), or over an extended period of multiple interviews in order to document their mental status and capabilities in relationship to the services to be provided.

It is important to always use a standardized form/questions in order to understand the client's emotional and cognitive processes. The MSE is not a separate, independent action, but is part of the overall intake process. Aside from general appearance, the Case Manager will note subtle visual and verbal clues about the client's thought process, impulse control, cognitive functioning and intelligence level, reality level and suicidal or homicidal tendencies. Active listening for both how and what the client says is important. Input from others is often necessary when the client either cannot provide information (e.g. about past events) or does not perform at an

intellectual level in order to communicate for themselves (due to chronological age or from the effects of their disease).

Long-term case management red flags

Long-term case management is usually determined by the diagnosis (e.g. multiple sclerosis, spinal cord injury, amputation, elderly end-of-life) and prognosis for cases requiring services for several months, years, or a lifetime. Red flags must be recognized and case management intervention initiated when an illness or treatment has a potential for long term treatment.

Red flags are often:
1) Lack of improvement, setbacks, or complications in routine cases
2) Terminal illness
3) Whenever treatment is 6 months or longer
4) Presence of multiple medical conditions
5) An increase in complications which is an indicator of possible systemic issues

CCM

CCM (Certified Case Manager) is an experience-based certification requiring a post-secondary degree in a field promoting the physical, psychosocial or vocational well-being of individuals that provides a license or certification to legally and independently practice that field without the supervision of another licensed professional. The license or certification must be current and active and the holder must be in good standing in the state in which they practice or by the credentialing body. In addition, applicants for CCM must satisfy one of the following:
- 12 months of acceptable, full-time, supervised case management experience documented by a Certified Case Manager

- 24 months of acceptable, full-time case management experience (no supervision requirement)
- 12 months of acceptable full-time case management employment experience as the supervisor of employees providing direct case management services

CCM certification qualifications

Since the CCM is an experience-based designation, the following must be part of the job description, or documented by the applicant's supervisor as part of their job responsibilities:

- Performance of all six essential activities of case management
- 5 out of 6 essential activities done directly with clients
- Consideration of the ongoing needs of the client across a continuum of care
- Services provided are interactive with relevant components of the client's healthcare system
- Consideration of the broad spectrum of the client's needs
- At least 50% of time is spent on
  - a) Direct case management
  - b) Supervision of those providing direct case management services
  - This provision requires submission of both your job description and the job description of the people you supervise

Case management core components

In order to qualify to be a Certified Case Manager, the essential activities of case management must be part of the individual's job tasks. These activities are assessment, planning, implementation, coordination, monitoring and evaluation.

The core components of case management are application of the six essential activities within the context of employment activities. The core components are:
1) Processes and relationships
2) Healthcare management
3) Community resources and support
4) Service delivery
5) Psychosocial intervention
6) Rehabilitation case management

The core components must be applied across a continuum of care at a level appropriate for the client's unique needs.

Vocational Concepts and Strategies

Managed care and managed competition

Managed Care Organization (MCO) is a generic term that is used to describe many types of medical care plans including HMO, PPO, IPA, etc. California's 1993 reforms for workers' compensation claims saw the creation of health care organizations (HCOs) to apply MCO principles to work-related injuries. As managed care evolves, dental care providers are creating managed care networks. Managed competition is the term given to the business environment created by the managed care entities competing for business. Many large companies are negotiating discount arrangements from healthcare and prescription providers, durable medical equipment supplies or rehabilitation facilities.

A Case Manager must be aware of the mergers taking place between providing companies to assure quality of care and the effects of business relationships on their ability to negotiate on behalf of their client. The Case Manager may also be limited in the offerings they can present in the individualized plan due to arrangements between the insurer and healthcare providers.

Raising status of their profession

Case management operates within a business community, thus Case Managers need to understand the business aspects of their profession and contribute to the marketing effort of their agency/company. Case Managers establish relationships with vendors and community businesses supplying goods and services to their clients; in many cases they are the only face and voice that the business connects with the agency.

Case Managers should present themselves as part of the solution to the nation's healthcare crisis. Submission of articles to professional journals and publications, membership in community and business groups, and interaction with healthcare leaders all contribute to elevating the status of Case Managers and spread an understanding of their contributions to healthcare. Case Managers should also contribute to their company/agency's effort to generate new business. The Case Manager has many referral contacts which should be shared with their marketing departments.

Case Manager background

Training alone does not create a good Case Manager. The work is complex, detailed, demanding and challenging. Success cannot be guaranteed, but the following personal characteristics and professional achievements increase the chances of succeeding in the field. Case management takes place in many different settings, so the professional background of the Case Manager can contribute to success. In a clinical setting, knowledge of medical procedures reduces the learning curve. Knowledge of alternative treatments and nontraditional settings is beneficial for successful case management in other settings.

Educational background, and continued education, contributes to the success of a Case Manager. Besides formal classes, knowledge is gained through workshops, conferences, and reading professional journals and newsletters. A Case Manager needs to be credible to her clients. Life experience provides an understanding of how to balance empathy and efficiency, when to negotiate and when to hold fast, and knowing when to push a client to use their own resources versus providing support. Personal qualities including a sense of humor, strong work ethic, believing that you can make a difference, and a sense of objectivity are important characteristics of a Case Manager.

CLAS standards

The CLAS standards are primarily directed at health care organizations; however, individual providers are also encouraged to use the standards to make their practices more culturally and linguistically accessible. The principles and activities of culturally and linguistically appropriate services should be integrated throughout an organization and undertaken in partnership with the communities being served.

The 14 standards are organized by themes:
- Culturally Competent Care (Standards 1–3)
- Language Access Services (Standards 4–7)
- Organizational Supports for Cultural Competence (Standards 8–14)

Within this framework, there are three types of standards of varying stringency: mandates, guidelines, and recommendations as follows:
- CLAS mandates are current federal requirements for all recipients of federal funds (Standards 4, 5, 6, and 7)
- CLAS guidelines are activities recommended by the Office of Minority Health (OMH) for adoption as mandates by federal, state, and national accrediting agencies (Standards 1, 2, 3, 8, 9, 10, 11, 12, and 13)

Culturally and Linguistically Appropriate Services (CLAS) in Health Care offered by the US Department of Health and Human Services Office of Minority Health National Standards.

Healthcare field changes

The latest trend in obtaining healthcare information is use of electronic technologies (e.g. the Internet) or e-health. This is providing patients with a plethora of information that both assists them in self-management and confuses them about care and treatment options.

Demand management is the concept of self-care case management through education of the patient so that they can determine potential problems and seek treatment when appropriate. E-health self-care is an important component of demand management. Case Managers are part of the decision trees in demand management scenarios and must make sure to fully document their interactions with patients.

The concept of 24-hour managed care coverage has received mixed reaction. Benefits include quick return-to-work time frames, economic and administrative savings through integration of the various insurance benefits available.

Alternatively, the 24-hour care scenario has legal, administrative and regulatory hurdles. Another emerging healthcare trend is the concept of "carving out" elements of a health plan to save costs. High volume and high cost treatments, as well as pharmaceutical, behavioral health and vision programs are often carved-out of the traditional health plan.

Worker's compensation case

Returning an employee to work is the goal of case management in worker's compensation claims. Early case management facilitates proper and timely medical care creates good public relations with employees, reduces the cost of health care, and aggressive case management reduces lost work time. Case Manager communication with providers facilitates a return to light-duty work or an adjustment in work requirements/atmosphere allowing return to work.

An overview of medical care provided by multiple sources prevents duplication of services. A Case Manager can assist in obtaining the highest quality of care as well as negotiate discounts and assist in containment of costs through appropriate physician selection. A Case Manager facilitates communication between all involved parties: employer, insurance adjustor, providers, employee and family.

Demand management

Demand management puts the burden of self-care on the patient. Case Managers provide education avenues to patients but need to make sure they do not assist in determination of a diagnosis. Patients will be looking for confirmation of the conclusions they have drawn, and Case Managers need to avoid this discussion and make sure to fully document their discussions with patients.

Case Managers must be aware of employers who use carve-out programs providing in-house resources (e.g. weight loss programs, on-site wellness activities). It is also important to know the employers utilizing outsourcing to achieve benefit oversight or customer service. The overseers of these carve-out programs and the outsource managers are contacts the Case Manager muse be aware of to provide assistance to their clients.

Case management growth areas

New solutions for healthcare challenges are sought by businesses, government, and insurers. Case Managers are posed to offer solutions and services. Public sector case management is growing with the goal of improving the quality of care, patient outcomes and reducing costs. Claims management is an area that can benefit clients as well as employers. Many elderly patients need medical bill audit assistance, along with claims management.

There have been cases of over billing and duplicate billing scams that would be caught with diligent oversight/management services. Many medical diagnoses can benefit from case management. Pregnancy management, wellness programs, prenatal, pediatric, elder care and disease-specific case management are areas of expansion for Case Managers. As home care become an option exercised more and more by patients, case management can play an important role.

Home care alternatives

Common alternatives to hospital treatment are rehabilitation and skilled nursing facilities. The newest alternative is home care, one of today's fastest growing industries, providing services by licensed/certified personnel in a setting that contributes to faster recovery, a better quality of life and decreased risk of contracting a nosocomial illness (an illness from a hospital-borne infection), all at substantial cost savings over formal facility care.

Home care is not for acutely ill individuals needing specialized programs or skilled nursing facilities. The family situation needs to be able to support the needs of the patient (treatment and medication schedules) without making them feel like a burden. Children improve quicker in a home setting with fewer lingering psychological issues. Technology has made it feasible to use home care for patients needing dialysis, blood transfusions, ventilators or pain management, as well long-term or illnesses such as AIDS, brain injury, or chronic neurological problems (multiple sclerosis) or those that are terminally ill. For patients recuperating from surgery, it is important to have a coordinated team approach to ensure that quality, comprehensive services are provided.

Case Managers for home care services

Coordination of services for home care is an important function of case management. Assuring the patient and family that home care is a viable, safe option is of primary importance, and then a visit to the home ensures home care can be accommodated. Liability for providing appropriate care is a function of all personnel involved in the patient's treatment plan; however the discharging, primary care physician must provide the sign off on discharge orders.

The Case Manager must devise a home care plan that meets all criteria of the discharge plan. The patient's family and community resources, geographical location and availability of health care and durable medical equipment providers as well as emergency services must be taken into account. Depending on the circumstances, Case Managers may need to make a case for coverage to the insurance carrier with cost savings as the primary benefit.

Case Manager's role
Home care is an area that requires detailed monitoring and documentation by Case Managers. Any deficiencies in performance of services by recommended

vendors reflect on the Case Manager and are subject to legal action. Input about vendor performance from the patient and care giver is important to obtain on a regular basis.

The Case Manager must be aware of changing needs of the patient and make sure they are reflected in the care plan. The patient's adherence to the care plan and successes or failures must be noted and adjustments made to the care plan to meet any changes. Care giver psychological and physical well being must also be noted and respite care investigated. Intervention with payers may be needed to cover respite care and the real threat of covering the costs of the care giver's breakdown is a compelling reason. It is important for the Case Manager to remember that their negotiation skills in obtaining cost effective services is the key to home health care savings. Their negotiation skills with the payer is also key in assuring that the cost of home care will be result in overall cost savings and thus be covered by the insurance plan, especially if a variance in coverage is needed.

Psychological, physical and emotional problems
Home care is not without drawbacks. The home must be able to accommodate the durable equipment needed and provide a safe environment for the patient for both recovery and treatment activities. A safe environment begins with the cleanliness of the home and the ability of the family to provide nourishment and cleanliness needed for healing. Often care givers need to use physical exertion to move patients. This can cause complications for the care giver as well as create an unsafe environment for patient.

The patient must have an environment that will allow healing and not make them feel like they are a burden to the care giver; the care giver cannot be in a position of feeling trapped into providing care. Case Managers must be cognizant throughout the case of stress on the care giver and the family and the resulting effect on the patient.

Resources for providing at-home services

Home care is available from a variety of sources. Skilled professionals in nursing and therapy fields are available through private sources, however cost savings are available by exploring alternative providers. Local, county or state agencies support a variety of professional services delivered in the home (e.g. visiting nurses association) or available at their facility on a day-visit basis (e.g. senior day care or dialysis). Disease-specific organizations (childhood diabetes), foundations and non-profit groups (Shiner's burn center) are also sources for home care support. Some of these same organizations offer respite care enabling the patient to spend up to a week away from home enabling the care giver to "recharge."

Respite care

Respite care is the psychological and physical support provided to care givers. Respite care takes many forms. Especially in cases involving long-term care, care givers need to be encouraged to talk with others in similar situations, facing similar challenges by attending care giver support groups. To better understand illnesses, support services are available for spouses, family and children/siblings of individuals suffering from long-term illnesses.

Respite care may be in the form of camp for a child suffering from an illness (cancer, diabetes) allowing the family to be free of responsibility for the time while the patient is away. Respite care may be placement of an elderly person at an assisted living residence for a weekend giving the family care providers a "week end off." Respite care may be someone residing in the home of a patient allowing the family care givers to take a vacation. Case Managers can assist by identifying when care givers need respite care and by supplying resources for respite care.

Assistance to families facing a crisis

Families of patients must deal with the effect of the patient on the normal operation of their family life. Realignment of family responsibilities occurs each time someone suffers from illness or injury, and prolonged illness puts unique burdens on the family dynamics. It is important for the Case Manager to understand the family dynamics and provide intervention resources when needed. If the family was fractured before the illness, changes are the fracture will intensify, causing problems in addressing the treatment plan of the patient. To assist families through periods of crisis, a Case Manager can suggest family counseling or support groups for the family or the care giver, recommend books on the illness or coping with illness, direct families to sources for financial assistance, remind the family that maintenance of their regular routines, appointments and activities is important to their physical and psychological health, and encourage the family to communicate with one another.

Ergonomics

Ergonomics is the study of the interaction of people and things, and designing and arranging them for efficient and safe interaction. Ergonomics has contributed to a healthy, productive, safer work environment. Case Managers have three

(3) areas for impact on ergonomics in the workplace:

1) The Case Manager may identify illnesses or injuries that occurred due to unsafe conditions on the job and report these to the appropriate company departments for further evaluation

2) When a job environment cannot be reasonable modified to accommodate a worker's limitations, the Case Manager may make referrals for strength or endurance training, work hardening, or vocational assessment or retraining

3) The Case Manager acts as an advocate for the worker making the employer aware of the worker's limitations and working with the employer to modify the work environment reduce work hours or responsibilities to allow lighter responsibilities during rehabilitation, or suggesting job-fit analysis to accommodate a permanently disabled worker.

Worker's Compensation

Worker's compensation provides coverage of injury or illness that occurs while an individual was at work or caused by a work-related task. The premiums are paid by the employer and the initial intent of the legislation was as an incentive for employers to increase worker's safety. Some benefits vary by state, however, payment of medical bills related to illness or injury or occupational diseases (e.g. black lung), as well as a percentage of lost wages is provided by Worker's Compensation.

There are also benefits in case of death and total or partial disability of the employee. If a worker is covered by and accepts coverage under Worker's Compensation, they may not claim benefits under a group insurance policy or bring suit against the employer for work-related injuries. It is very important for Case Managers to have documentation in the individual's plan if the case is being handled through Worker's Compensation.

Work hardening program

Work hardening programs are individualized, multidisciplinary therapy programs designed to return workers to full employment. Work hardening programs use real or work-simulated activities along with conditioning exercises and psychosocial treatments to address the patient's ability to return to work. They do not treat the underlying condition that led to the disability nor are they designed to return the patient to independent living. Once the patient is sufficient recovered to participate in the process, work hardening programs are suitable for patients who have a job and whose therapy can be related to their return to work, the physical, psychological and vocational deficits can be documented, and the patient is willing to participate in the therapy.

Case Management Principles and Strategies

Conflicts of interest in a client/manager relationship

Dual relationship is when you have a relationship with the client outside your role as Case Manager (e.g. family member, friend, and co-worker). Favoritism, asking a client for a favor (e.g. haircut, manicure, child care), can put you in a position where the client can request a favor in return. Acceptance of gifts from clients should only be done under the spirit of accepting for the office (e.g. candy at a holiday). Sexual and romantic relationships must always be avoided.

If the client's problem involves religious, moral, political or ethical issues, values conflict could prohibit your ability to provide unbiased services. Recognize these value conflicts and request assistance from someone else in your office.

Informed consent

All clients have the right to consent to or withdraw from services. Agency policies about consent must be made clear during the intake process. Presentation of treatment or service options must include a discussion of possible side effects, risks, consequences, and benefits of treatment, medications, or procedures, including consequences or risks of stoppage of the service. The capacity of the client to make clear, competent decisions must be taken into account when providing clear and easy to understand information of what is included in the treatment, as well as alternate procedures that are available.

Check for comprehension of the information by asking appropriate questions. Consent must be self-determined; it is imperative that the client has not been coerced or pressured by the agency or the provider of the service. Once information has been provided verbally and in writing, a signed consent form must be retained in the case management records.

Release of HIV/AIDS information

A blanket release of information form is not sufficient when dealing with HIV/AIDS information. Most states require a signed form specifically stating permission is granted to release the client's HIV status. Without specific state requirements, you are still responsible for protecting your client and should involve the client in a discussion about release of potentially harmful information.

Documentation of the discussion should be part of the client's records. If written permission is not obtained in states with requirements for a form, all reference to the client's HIV status must be deleted, including information about any testing and whether or not it was negative or positive.

Guarding confidentiality of clients

Clients need to grant permission for their information to be shared, whether this sharing is with colleagues, healthcare professionals, schools, or agency personnel. The agency may have a release form in addition to their standard HIPAA form. Anyone who has access to client information must sign a confidentiality agreement.

Never talk about cases, even with the names omitted. Information cannot be shared as part of a teaching situation with students or interns, unless the participants have signed confidentiality agreements. Never acknowledge that someone is a client. Agencies have procedures for handling requests for information that must be followed.

Review a client's request for release of information and assist those who are impaired in their decision-making capacity on what information is considered confidential. Confidentiality must be followed in the releasing information to schools as it could prejudice future decisions about a child.

Breaking client confidentiality circumstances

Confidentiality can be broken in the following circumstances:
- To protect others from possible harmful actions by the client. Notification of intent to harm should be provided to the other party as well as the police
- To provide emergency services to the client, e.g. providing information to the emergency room about the medicine consumed
- To protect clients from inflicting harm on themselves
- To notify authorities of suspected abuse, neglect, exploitation, births, and suspicious deaths
- To report specific diseases as required by public health laws
- To comply with a court order or subpoena
- To obtain payment for services. The agency would refer a client for non-payment only after reasonable attempts to collect the payment has been made and if the client has made no effort to arrange for even minimal payment

- To obtain a professional consultation regarding how to best proceed with a case

HIPAA's relationship to case management

Title II of HIPAA (Health Insurance Portability and Accountability Act) contains the rules for protecting a client's health information. The act covers not only formal records, but also personal notes and billing information. HIPAA covers release of protected health information (PIH) released, transferred, or divulged outside the agency. It was instituted due to the request from insurance companies for client information.

The agency's HIPAA form must be in plain, understandable language and include the agency's privacy and confidentiality procedures. The form must include to whom the information might be released and the purpose for releasing the information. It must be signed and dated by the client and have an expiration date.

Information released under HIPAA becomes protected under the confidentiality guidelines of the organization receiving the information. The agency must have a privacy officer and safeguards to protect client records. The safeguards include electronic security of files (e.g. passwords) and security of work areas and destruction of files/information.

Privileged communication

Privileged communication protects the right of a client to withhold information in a court proceeding. Privileged communication is a legal term for a right that belongs to the client. State law specifically states the professionals who are considered recipients of privileged communications. A client waives their right to privileged communication if they sue the agency or if they use their condition as a defense in a legal proceeding. You must turn over certain information if so mandated by a court, or if you are acting in a court-appointed capacity, e.g. guardian or payee.

Information about clients can be shared to protect clients and those connected with them from harm. These circumstances include intent to commit suicide, commit a crime, harm another person, a need to be hospitalized for a mental condition, or when a child under 16 may be the victim of a sexual or physical abuse situation.

Client record security

Agency/company policies regarding record security must be in place and regularly reviewed with staff. Electronic records need to be limited to those with a "need to know." This is accomplished by restricting access via passwords, an audit trail showing file access, secure placement of any equipment (computers, printers, and faxes), appropriate backup and storage procedures, encrypted files, and firewalls on networks.

Paper records should always be secured and a reference to file number or patient codes used as opposed to use of names. Paper shredders should always be used; realize that telephone messages including names and phone numbers must be protected. Locks on doors, files, and brief cases must always be engaged. Release of information should not be done without checking for the written client release or waiver. Only explicitly requested information is communicated. Check with the security officer or legal counsel before releasing sensitive information (e.g. HIV/AIDS, substance abuse, and medical condition); every agency/company should have a security officer/designate.

Violation of medical privacy

At companies with more than 25 employees, inquiries about medical information or requiring a physical exam cannot be done prior to an offer of employment. Denial of a job based on a physical examination can only be done if the "essential functions" of that job cannot be performed (e.g. cannot lift up to 50 pounds for an employee of a shipping company).

Redress is available under Title I and V of the Americans with Disabilities Act of 1990 which prohibits employment discrimination against qualified individuals in state, local or private sector jobs. Sections 501 and 505 of the Rehabilitation Act of 1973 prohibit employment discrimination against qualified individuals in federal government employment. The Civil Rights Act of 1991 provides monetary damages in international employment discrimination.

Ethical duties/legal duties

Legal duties are described by a society as minimum acceptable standards of conduct. Failure to perform a legal duty up to standards usually carries a punishment.

Ethics are rules or standards governing the conduct of a person or members of a profession. Ethical duties are ideal conduct for an individual or professional, as determined by the society. Ethical conduct that does not meet the standards and is not illegal is only punishable by the professional society.

As a rule, ethical duties usually exceed those of legal duties. In the case of conflict between legal and ethical duties, the American Medical Association (AMA) holds that the ethical duties supersede the legal duties.

Ethical principles

Five ethical principles of case management are:
1) The patient's autonomy is the freedom to choose his own treatment path. Through the use of education and empowerment the patient will be self-directed
2) The Case Manager must exhibit beneficence (being kind and charitable), acting as the patient's advocate, doing good for the patient, rather than for herself, the provider or the insurer
3) By actively seeking to prevent harm from coming to the patient, the Case Manager exhibits nonmalfeasance. This is accomplished via education and counseling
4) The concept of justice is demonstrated by ensuring equity of treatment for one's patients. Healthcare treatment will be allocated based on individual needs. Being just or fair must balance what is best for one's patient versus what is just for the larger society
5) Adhering to the truth and establishing rapport is veracity. It is the obligation of the Case Manager to deal factually, truthfully and accurately, establishing a trusting relationship with the patient and others

Ethical decision making

The Case Manager has the obligation to act in the best interest of the patient, the payer and society at large. Clashes and conflict will occur in serving these parties, as well as by the ethical dilemma when two or more equally desirable outcomes are in conflict and only one outcome is possible:
- Deciding which of the equally desirable outcomes will occur is often the job of the Case Manager
- The selection of one outcome implies that the other outcomes will not occur
- The beneficiaries of the outcomes not selected will be displeased and may feel alienated or betrayed by the Case Manager
- The Case Manager must acknowledge that the decision that was made was the most fair and mindful given the situation, thus reinforcing that the Case Manager made an ethical decision. Without this realization, the Case Manager will suffer self doubt and decision paralysis.

Case Management dilemmas

There are three common dilemmas in Case Management. Discuss each type:
- Focus of advocacy is the conflict faced by the Case Manager between the best interests of the patient, the patient's family, the payer and society at large. An example is a terminal ill patient in need of expensive treatment who has reached the end of their insurance coverage with a family having no financial resources and strong religious convictions regarding end-of-life options.
- Supremacy of values becomes a problem when there is a clash between the values held by the Case Manager, the Case Manager's employer, the patient or their family, or the insurer. Determining whose value should

reign supreme in making decisions has no right answer.

- Conflict of duties occurs when a Case Manager, in carrying out the wishes of their client, may cause harm to others. This often occurs in maintaining the confidentiality of the patient's condition, e.g. HIV status

Patient assessment importance

The Case Manager has a responsibility to provide a comprehensive assessment of the patient's medical, intellectual, educational, psychological, social, religious and financial status. Without an intimate understanding of the patient, a Case Manager's recommendations may lead to disastrous outcomes due to unrecognized barriers to care. The assessment is part of the patient's file and admissible in court if a suit is filed.

Prepared assessment forms assist in gathering all needed information and should include, at a minimum, chief complaint, current diagnoses, current treatments including medications and the treatment plan, past medical history, social history including education level, family and community support system, sexual history and orientation, history of substance abuse, religious affiliations and involvement, insurance eligibility, private and federal programs, the client's benefits package, and the expected outcomes of the case.

Ostensible agency and negligent referrals

When the Case Manager makes referrals to specific providers, then under the law, the providers become an "agent" of the Case Manager; an ostensible agency relationship is established. Due to this relationship, negligent actions taken by the provider draw the Case Manager into subsequent litigation. Negligent referral occurs when the Case Manager refers a patient to a healthcare provider who is known to be unqualified due to a lack of skill or judgment.

The Case Manager must be knowledgeable about the provider's licensure, accreditation, certifications, relevant clinical experience and any history of patient complaints, malpractice or criminal activity. The lack of skill or judgment may be due to physical or mental impairment caused by drug abuse or alcoholism, or due to general carelessness or apathy. The Case Manager should reference the qualifications of referred providers as opposed to their quality. Recommending several providers allows the patient to make the decision. The Case Manager should follow up with patients to review their experience with providers and take appropriate action to report dissatisfaction, negligence or misconduct.

Tort

Tort is from the Latin torquere and means injury, damage, or a wrongful act done willfully, negligently, or in situations involving strict liability committed against a person or property without the need for physical contact. Tort feasor is the person who is legally accountable for the damage caused.

Due diligence

Due diligence is the effort made by someone to avoid harming himself or someone else. It is often used in a contract specifying someone will provide due diligence. Failure results in negligence.

Competence

Competence is the mental ability and capacity to make decisions, perform actions and tasks based upon the adequate performance of others with a similar background and training.

COBRA

The Consolidated Omnibus Reconciliation Act created COBRA as a means to allow an employee who leaves a company to continue on their company's health insurance plan for a specified period of time thus avoiding a lapse in coverage.

Indemnity

Indemnity refers to a traditional insurance plan where payment is made for loss or personal injury based on a contract. The contract of benefits and entitlements is paid by premiums made by an individual or company.

Abandonment

Abandonment is the termination of a professional relationship (e.g. physician/patient) resulting in injury to the patient because there was not sufficient notice to the patient or the opportunity for the patient to arrange for alternative care or services.

Bill of Particulars

Bill of Particulars is elaboration of a legal complaint providing more details and detailing more information in order to clarify the claim against the person.

Comparative Negligence

Comparative Negligence is method of measuring negligence shared among each person named in a suit, whether defense or plaintiff. Damages are reduced in proportion to the amount of negligence attributed to the complaining party.

Res ipsa loquitor

Res ipsa loquitor is the principle of law applied to cases where proof that something took place shifts the burden of proof to the defendant who must prove that the situation was not caused by the defendant's negligence. Implied is the defendant had exclusive control of the situation and the situation would not normally occur if the defendant's negligence had not been present. An example is leaving a surgical instrument in the patient following a surgical procedure (assuming a single surgeon was involved). Latin: The thing speaks for itself.

Agency

Agency is the principal/agent relationship between two or more persons where the principal allows the agent to act on his behalf. This is the relationship between the Case Manager and her employer and often results in a conflict of interest due to the Case Manager's obligations to her employers and the professional duties she owes her patient.

The Case Manager, in representing her employer must use care and skill, act in good faith, stay within the limits of the agent's authority, and obey the principal by acting solely for the principal's benefit, carrying out all reasonable instructions and advancing the interests of the principal.

Corporate Negligence

This term comprises the legal grounds for managed care organizations' liability based on the corporate activities of the organization as opposed to the care-related activities of the involved healthcare providers. Examples of corporate negligence is negligent credentialing, failure to exercise

- 31 -

reasonable care in screening and selecting providers or staff, or negligent supervision, or failure to exercise reasonable oversight during the relationship with providers or staff.

Respondeat Superior

The principal is liable for the wrongful actions of his agent. A hospital can be held liable for the wrongful actions of the doctors or nurses its employs. A Case Manager may be held liable due to negligent actions of a provider when an ostensible agency relationship exists, e.g. the client was directed to only a single provider. Latin: Let the master answer.

Ex Parte

A legal proceeding, order, injunction, etc. brought about or granted by one party and to benefit of that party only, without notice to, or contestation by, any person adversely interested.

Fiduciary

A relationship where one person acts in another's best interest. This special relationship is usually based on trust, confidence or responsibility and encompasses a trustee, guardian, counselor, institution or a volunteer.

Validity

Validity is the probability that the practices will lead to the projected outcomes.

TEFRA

TEFRA is the Tax Equity and Fiscal Responsibility Action of 1982. In order to provide incentives for cost containment, this legislation established:
- Diagnosis Related Groups (DRGs) determining the cost of care for

selected diagnosis and placed limits on rate increases in hospital revenues
- Exempted medical rehabilitation from DRGs maintaining it as cost-based reimbursement system
- Made employer group health plans for employees 65 to 69 and their spouses in that age group superior to Social Security and Medicare
- Revised the Age Discrimination in Employment Act (ADEA) of 1967 requiring employers to offer the same health benefits to active employees aged 65 to 69 and their spouses as those offered to younger employees
- Established Peer Review Organizations (PROs) for Medicare and Medicaid patients to ensure adequate treatment while reducing costs associated with hospital stays and also to conduct reviews of their hospital-based care to ensure quality of care and appropriateness of admissions, readmissions, and discharges

Mental Health Parity Action of 1996

Protecting individuals with mental health problems, the MHPA prohibits lifetime or annual dollar limits on mental healthcare, unless the same limits apply to medical or surgical treatment. MHPA exempts employers with 50 or fewer employees, or if requirements will result in significant hardship, specifically an increase of 1% or more in its healthcare costs. The key aspects are:
- Exclusion of chemical dependency is allowed as well as allowing separate limits for treatment of substance abuse
- Plans can still exclude mental health treatment, but if included, they cannot have separate dollar limits from medical care

Although annual or lifetime dollar limits cannot be set, the following are allowed:

- limited number of annual outpatient visits and annual inpatient days
- per-visit fee limits
- higher deductibles and co-payments for mental health benefits than for medical and surgical treatment

Pregnancy Discrimination Act

An individual cannot be discriminated against in regard to choice, access, cost and quality of treatment in maternity benefits when compared with medical benefits. The enforcement is independent of the marital status of the employee. This includes health insurance benefits, short-term sick leave, disability benefits and employment policies dealing with seniority, leave extensions and reinstatement.

The following categories of employees are eligible under the Pregnancy Discrimination Act:

- full and part time employees
- independent contractors
- employees of successor corporations
- employees of parent-subsidiary groups

Abortions and mandatory maternity leave are not covered under the Act. Private employers with fewer than fifteen employees are exempt.

Prevent malpractice suits

Prevention of malpractice suites includes the following:

- Be honest and open with clients; ensure you have clear and concise informed consent procedures and never promise what you cannot deliver
- Make sure your contracts define the Case Manager's role as one providing help or assistance to their clients'
- Make sure fees are clearly defined in your contract
- Abandonment is a key malpractice suit so be sure to provide coverage when you are unavailable to your clients (sickness or vacation)
- Maintain detailed documentation of treatment plans and up-to-date and accurate records of clients
- Be aware of agency policies where you work as well as local, state and federal laws; be involved in professional organizations to ensure you keep up-to-date
- Remember to obtain written consent whenever client information needs to be shared or you will be working with minors; know the laws when confidential information must be communicated to other health or protective agencies.
- Remember to always display courtesy working with clients and behave in an ethical manner; work within the policies of the agency/company where you are employed
- Find sources for consultation or supervision and use them when unsure of the actions to take or for potential legal or ethical situations
- Monitor your clients and make sure they know how to evaluate their progress toward their goals

Documenting a case file

Always be aware of local and state laws for documentation that you prepare or reimbursement for services may be withheld. The following should always be followed:

- use black ink; never use pencil
- do not use correction fluid
- make all notes legible
- remember confidentiality rules in identifying the client on each page; date of birth for children's records is often required
- always put the date of the client contact
- sign every note (no initials)
- put the date the note was written after your signature
- end notations with the next appointment or follow up date
- correct mistakes my drawing a line through the error and write "error" and sign or initial and date the error note
- draw a line through any blank lines on the page (so that no information can be added later)

Positive communications with physicians

Focused and conscious communications between Case Managers and physicians must be established and maintained. It is important for Case Managers to use medical terminology in their communications with physicians and for the physician to realize the Case Manager can provide education and support services to their patients. Often the Case Manager role is not understood by physicians since they are brought into the case after initial treatment has started.

Physicians often lack insight into the social and environmental aspects of the patient; Case Managers provide this insight. Power struggles occasionally occur in care planning since decisions by physicians are often made from a different agenda then Case Managers; the Case Manager's role must be made clear to the physician. Physicians may not be aware of limited policy coverage or lack of community support once discharge takes place. Case Managers provide this information and assist in the discharge or care plan creation.

Case Manager's report

Initial and subsequent Case Manager Reports need to sell the management plan and its role in problem solving, outline the cost savings due to case management, and address any anticipated objectives available due to creative, analytical thinking. The interest of the patient must predominate. The report must present an objective view while meeting the unique requirements of the entity receiving the document. Besides containing the main points for the reason the client came into the Case Manager's load, the report must contain information about the payer source(s), medical history and current physicians, a review of policy coverage and limitations, and community resources and alternative treatment programs.

Make sure all recommendations are presented as to their ability to meet the patient's needs and present provider information about their quality of services and ability to meet patient needs. A presentation on the costs of treatment should be included in a separate section so it does not appear as an influence to recommended services.

Utilization reviews

Utilization reviews evaluate the need for services, the appropriateness of the services and the efficiency of those services. The reviews should support the need for the continuance or discontinuance of actions or interventions.

Preadmission review allows documentation for the need for case management (3-5% of cases), rather than just acting as a census tool. It catches the unique aspect of each case and begins building the red flags needing resolution so that the case proceeds smoothly (e.g. notification to payer).

Concurrent review shows the success or failure of treatments and provides the data for reducing lengths of stay or exploring alternative care plans. Concurrent review also documents the required processes for discharge success.

Retrospective review allows the Case Manager to support their role in the treatment plan and provides valuable information in planning future, similar cases.

Cost-benefit analysis reports

Attaching value to the job of a Case Manager is an important aspect of their role. Case management adds cost to a program, but costs that are, hopefully, offset by savings. At a minimum, cost-benefit reports should contain an overview and summary of case management intervention, any fees attached to the case management tasks, actual charges and the savings, both gross and net, and the status of the case being reported. Potential savings should be documented and although they are difficult to quantify, these segments of the case need to be included in order to present a complete picture of the case.

When a Case Manager works for a client (HMO or self-insured employer), it is recommended that a cost-benefit analysis of their case load is submitted every quarter. Quarterly reporting allows a manageable amount of information to be processed and the effectiveness of services to be reviewed on a timely basis

that allows for adjustments to the plans, if necessary. Be aware that cost-benefit analysis reports are often used by the marketing and quality assurance departments of organizations.

End of services survey

At the conclusion of a case, especially an involved or long-term relationship case, it is important to provide the client with a satisfaction survey. The survey or questionnaire must be as objective as possible. The survey results assure clients that case management does make a difference to the families receiving the services. The results affirm that the services provided are those needed by the recipients of the services. Responses are a tool used to train professionals, meet the needs of patients, and respond to the expectations of payers. The public relations and marketing departments also appreciate the results of user surveys.

Long-term care cases

A payers' relationship with the Case Manager is important for smooth implementation of long-term cases. Honesty with the payer is very important including communication of patient setbacks. The level of involvement of a Case Manager is dependent on the patient's medical history, age, diagnosis, current medical situation, treatment plan and required services, family and community support, timing of receiving the case, and the patient's benefit plan.

Benefits of case management are early identification of a possible long-term case to document services needed and implement cost controls, cost containment, presentation of findings to the referral source, improvements in the situation due to case management, presence of an objective and encouraging attitude with the patient and family, and identification of an end goal, where improvement provides positive encouragement and terminal illness indicates more stressful cases.

Challenges

Long-term care is characterized by long periods of slow, insignificant progress or plateaus, and the hurdles of dealing with changing providers and possibly Case Managers. Changes in providers causes stress for both the patient and their family and can cause a temporary setback.

Case Managers need to reestablish their relationship with the new providers to provide patient information. Long term cases often incur complications including short-term illness, degradation of the primary condition or introduction of new diagnoses which change the treatment plan. Changing family or home care situations also impact the treatment plan.

Aging parents may indicate the need for transfer of patient services from the home to a facility. The financial burden of a long-term illness requires review of the patient and/or family's finances on a regular basis.

Financial burden

Long-term cases place a financial burden on the families and the payers. It is important for Case Managers to make sure these cases are not prematurely closed. Long-term cases provide a situation requiring smart negotiation skills by the Case Manager. A long-term case guarantees income to the providers and presents an opportunity for the Case Manager to negotiate a reduced rate for a long-term contract.

Conversely, once an established case becomes long-term or the need for services change, the Case Manager should renegotiate the vendor's rate to benefit the payer and the family. (This cost-containment measure is important to capture in the Case Manager's report.) To assist families in dealing with the financial burden of long-term case care, the Case Manager may need to supply information on alternative funding sources (public or private) and assist with applications for aide.

Public sector case management

Public sector case management includes those patients on Medicare and Medicaid. Intervention and case management is targeted for high-risk pregnancy, high-risk newborns, sickle cell anemia, AIDS, psychiatric, cancer and drug and alcohol patients. Working with this population presents challenges since there is often a lack of access to financial and transportation resources in order for the clients to help themselves.

Public sector individuals may have easier access to out-of-plan solutions since the system is flexible and review and approval by a payer is not required. A challenge for Case Managers is finding providers who will accept Medicaid payment, which is significantly lower than what private providers pay for services. The population also presents a challenge because elderly patients have multiple medical challenges, may be confused by the delivery system and associated processes, and due to financial restraints, may not take medications as prescribed. An additional challenge is that support services to prevent complications from Alzheimer's disease are not covered.

Good communication barriers

Five barriers to good communication are as follows:
- Physical interference occurs when the client is distracted by the physical surroundings. Optimum

communications occurs in a quiet space without distractions

- Psychological noise occurs when the client is thinking about something else. This could be pain, hunger, anger or the issue of payment for services. Be sure the client is as comfortable as possible and explain that services are part of their benefit package and no additional cost
- Information overload is caused by an abundance of information or cognitive, intellectual or educational deficits. Notice the client's eye contact, ask questions to assess the client's understanding, and use vocabulary the client understands
- Perceptual barriers block your message or filter the information. These occur based on the client's unique experiences, cultural background, education level, or value system
- Structural barriers are caused by layers of bureaucracy or communication the client or their family deals with. Written communication between the clinical team and client insures clarity for all involved

Successful negotiation

Conflict in desires or needs between two or more people requires negotiation to reach a mutually satisfactory resolution. Case Managers will often negotiate on behalf of their clients with insurance companies or providers of services, the goals of both parties' need to be met.

A successful negotiation occurs within a reasonable timeframe and without excess expense. The ability of both parties to comply with the agreement, as well as the predictable changes over time, are necessary for a successful negotiation to be workable and enduring. A successful negotiation does not necessarily mean all parties are happy with the outcome, however, an agreement made within minimum time and expense that meets the true interests of the parties establishes a basis of clear communication that fosters an environment for future, successful negotiations.

A workable agreement allows both parties to meet their obligations within the time allotted. An enduring agreement has the ability to function successfully over the term of the agreement with enough flexibility to accommodate the variability of the patient's health, finances and family situation.

Unsuccessful negotiation

The outcome of an unsuccessful negotiated settlement might have a won/lost result. "Getting the best of the other party" or "taking them to the cleaners" does not facilitate honest communication in future dealings.

Persons or groups that feel they have been taken advantage of during negotiations may exhibit a lack of cooperation, anger and inflexibility in future negotiations, even if the point of contention is minor and easily solved. Preconceived negative attitudes between the parties and with the Case Manager are established. Unsuccessful negotiations will not present future opportunities. Dealing with a vendor for one client may pave the way for others to also benefit only if the negotiation is successful.

Successful negotiation factors

Information is one key to successful negotiation; know the important factors for each circumstance. Keep focused on the patient. Remember BATNA: "best

- 37 -

alternative to a negotiated agreement." This allows the Case Manager to explore alternate solutions rather than persisting in a negotiation that will not provide a desirable result. Both parties must trust the negotiator. Trust is built via good, timely communication and rapid action at times of agreement. Respect involves taking into consideration all parties involved in the negotiation, setting times and deliverables in a manner to takes into account everyone's' schedules and circumstances.

Avoid "irritators" during discussions. Irritators are terms that are judgmental or cause pain or embarrassment to either party, during negotiations state specifics and facts without emotion or personal qualifiers.

Active listening skills are essential to successful negotiations. Active listening includes understanding what is said, thinking about the content and implications of what is said. Active listening includes direct and indirect communications, e.g. body language, facial expressions, tone and nuances of speech. Repetition of major points not only shows you have been actively listening, but clarifies the content and meaning of the discussion and allows exploration of possible alternatives.

Patient advocate

Acting as patients' advocate is the primary role of the Case Manager. The need for a Case Manager comes from physical and emotional effects of the disease process or as a result of being overwhelmed by the quantity and complexity of the treatment plan.

The Case Manager assists the patient and his family to attain self-determination and autonomy by empowering them with education about their disease, clarifying available options and services, explaining insurance benefits, community resources, and listening. The Case Manager has a legal and ethical responsibility to protect patients from misinformation and errors in comprehension. The Case Manager can obtain more information or clarification from providers. The Case Manager can also help the patient clarify their needs or wishes to their family and caregivers. The Case Manager has a major role in ensuring the patient's wishes are documented and observed.

Malpractice suits

To avoid a malpractice suit in dealing with patient discharge, change in treatment placement or denial of services, Case Managers must aggressively seek all data necessary to make an informed decision. Case Managers must balance patient needs, payers limits (both monetary and pre-determined illness plans), and availability of facilities within the context of the best interests of the patient.

The easiest way to decrease the risks involved with patient discharges is thorough review of the patient's medical record, discuss the intention to discharge with the patient and the treating physician, confirm the adequacy of follow-up medical care, and confirm the patient's social support network. Physicians have the primary responsibility for the welfare of the patient and cannot shift responsibility of premature discharge or denial of service to the payer without documenting their protest of the payer's decision (Wickline v. State of California). The decisions must be documented by the Case Manager. Letters of denial must contain all the information needed to appeal the decision, including explanation of the appeals process and timelines.

Risks of litigation

Bad faith claims often stem from the perception of inappropriate denial of benefits. Bad faith occurs when there is no reasonable basis for the denial of benefits and the insurer is aware of this as the reason for the denial, or the insurer's complicated, unnecessary or tangled bureaucracy causes delays in approval of procedures. Case Managers should always:

- Have the Medical Director issue claims denials which are based upon documented procedures for determining medical necessity
- Document all rational for denial of services
- perform a thorough review of medical records documenting the time, date and findings of the review
- Consult legal counsel or medical experts, if necessary, in determining benefit allowance and exclusions
- Be aware of regulatory and contractual turnaround times for reviewing cases and complete within 24 hours if the timeline is not defined and inform the subscriber if the review will take longer
- If treatment is denied, the Case Manager should inform the subscriber of the appeals process, including the name and contact information of the appeals coordinator

Full disclosure and informed consent

A patient has the right to control the course of his own medical treatment. Full disclosure means presenting all of the facts needed to make a decision intelligently, within the intellectually ability of the patient or their representative.

Informed consent must be given voluntarily. The patient must have the capacity to give consent and be an adult (or have consent given by their legal guardian), consent must be given before a professional relationship is established and must be documented.

Full disclosure for treatment or a medical intervention means the patient has received a full description along with the projected or desired outcomes of the proposed treatment, therapy or surgery/procedure. The patient understands the likelihood of the success of the treatment and reasonably understands the risks or hazards inherent in the proposed treatment. The patient has been provided alternatives to the proposed care or treatment plan and understands the consequences of foregoing the treatment. Informed consent is required by law and lack of full disclosure constitutes assault and battery.

Malpractice risk management

Malpractice litigation can arise from a breach of obligation: the failure to do something that should be done - omission, or by doing something that should not be done - commission. The person who sues (plaintiff) must provide two points: negligence on the part of the Case Manager and injury resulting from the negligence, with injury being the key to the case.

Case Managers should practice the following management practices to minimize the risk of malpractice suits:

- utilize credentialed, reputable providers
- offer several choices of providers, if possible
- be consistent in decision making using written guidelines if possible

- document justification when varying from written criteria
- document patient discussions noting the patient's participation in the decision process
- document the patient's compliance in the treatment plan
- establish quality assurance programs to ensure consistency in decision-making and payment guidelines
- implement grievance procedures adhering to state guidelines for timeliness
- address the patient's concerns and be in contact with the patient's physician

NMHPA

The Newborns' and Mothers' Health Protection Act of 1996 (NMHPA) was enacted to cover hospital lengths of stay following childbirth. The law applies to both private and public employers. Nonfederal government and self-insured insurance plans can elect to "opt out" of this requirement under NMHPA. Under NMHPA, group health plans and health insurance issuers may not:
- restrict the length of hospital stays or require advance authorization for the stays for vaginal births to less than 48 hours or less than 96 hours for delivery by cesarean section
- increase an individual's coinsurance related to the 48 or 96 hour hospital stay
- deny coverage under the insurance plan solely to avoid NMHPA
- provide rebates or monetary compensation to a mother to encourage her to accept less than the minimum NMHPA protections
- penalize in any way an attending provider who provides care to a mother or newborn under NMHPA protections
- provide monetary or other incentives to an attending provider in order to persuade the provider to furnish care in a manner inconsistent with the NMHPA coverage

Pregnancy Discrimination Act

The Pregnancy Discrimination Act is an amendment to Title VII of the Civil Rights Act of 1964 stating pregnancy, childbirth or related medical conditions must be treated the same for employment-related purposes, e.g. coverage by insurance and the same job protections for any other type of illness.

MHPA

The Mental Health Parity Act (MHPA) required insurance plans to apply similar aggregate lifetime and annual dollar limits on mental health benefits as those applied to medical/surgical benefits whenever a plan included mental health benefits. It does not require mental health benefits be offered as part of the plan. If a plan has no limits on medical/surgical benefits, there cannot be limits on mental health benefits. MHPA is not applicable to benefits for substance or chemical dependency.

WHCRA

The Women's Health and Cancer Rights Act (WHCRA) requires insurance coverage of breast reconstruction or complications of mastectomy if the plan provided medical and surgical benefits for the mastectomy.

Legislation and its impact

Taft-Hartley Act
Taft-Hartley Act in the 1950s allowed the establishment of multi-employer benefit trusts thus providing healthcare coverage for union employees who work for more than one employer. The trust is overseen by both union and employer representatives.

Wickline v. State of California
Wickline v. State of California found that Case Managers are liable for damages if their referral of patients to providers is carelessly done and the patient is harmed as a direct result of the referral. This means Case Managers must make sure care givers or vendors meet standards set by various governing boards and accreditation groups.

Warne v. Lincoln National Administrative Services Corp
Warne v. Lincoln National Administrative Services Corp., based on the tenets of veracity, found the insurance company at fault because their literature did not plainly state policy exclusions thus the denial of benefits was done in bad faith. The benefit plan policy did not cover liver transplants, however, the benefit brochure listed organ transplants as a covered procedure, and thus misleading the consumer to believe the liver transplant would be covered by the plan.

Nazay v. Miller
Nazay v. Miller determined a patient must assume some responsibility for not meeting a health plan's requirements, e.g. if the plan administrator is not informed of the individual's hospitalization, the plan does not need to pay the full expenses incurred (payment is based on the plan's policy for covering non-approved health expenses).

Wilson v. Blue Cross of So. Calif. and Alabama and Western Medical Review
Wilson v. Blue Cross of So. Calif. and Alabama and Western Medical Review re-enforced the Wickline decision by affirming that when an organization substantially shapes the course of patient care, they can be held liable for the quality of the care received.

McClellan v. Health Maintenance Organization of Pennsylvania
McClellan v. Health Maintenance Organization of Pennsylvania held that a managed care organization could be held liable for injuries that results from a poor selection of doctors as members of the HMO network. The court reasoned that the HMO had what is called a nondelegable duty to verify the qualifications/quality of its primary care providers and only retain those that are competent. (This is similar to the responsibility of the Case Manager in suggesting care providers to its clients (Wickline v. California).

Linthicum v. Nationwide Life Insurance Company
Linthicum v. Nationwide Life Insurance Company states that in order to obtain punitive damages against an insurance company, clear and convincing evidence must be presented that shows the insurer consciously disregarded the fact that its conduct would injure or cause a substantial risk of harm to the insured.

Drolet v. Healthsource
Drolet v. Healthsource found that the HMO (Healthsource) must act with good faith, fair dealing, loyalty, candor, and full and fair disclosure. The case also cites a conflict of interest for doctors and company personnel who:
- own Healthsource stock
- have involvement in key decision making about guidelines and treatment

- retain the ability to terminate physicians without cause

California Psychological Assn. v. AETNA State Care Health Plan

California Psychological Assn. v. AETNA State Care Health Plan found that an insurance carrier cannot make care decisions, e.g. limiting services, rather than allowing the recommendations of the attending healthcare professionals. The insurance carrier wanted to replace psychotherapy with limited crisis intervention. This case demonstrates the need for detailed treatment plans that support the recommended services.

Bergalis v. CIGNA Dental Health Plan

Bergalis v. CIGNA Dental Health Plan spurred discussion of the problem of confidentiality when a practitioner has AIDs and the policies that need to be put into place to protect his patients.

Hughes v. Blue Cross of No. Calif.

Hughes v. Blue Cross of No. Calif. ruled that insurance companies cannot deny coverage when a physician has ordered hospitalization. If denial is done, it must be substantiated in written form and only after thorough review of all the patient's current and past medical history.

Examination before trial

Examination before trial is also referred to as "discovery." This allows lawyers to review facts and documents to prepare for trial.

Hold harmless

Hold harmless is usually part of a settlement agreement where one party agrees to pay any costs or claims. These claims would occur from the original situation.

Liability

Liability refers to the legal responsibility of someone's acts or omissions. Failure to meet the responsibility can result in a lawsuit.

Summons

Summons is a document issued to defendants following the filing of a lawsuit. The summons will state all the particulars of the lawsuit and a time limit for responding to the summons.

Subpoena

Subpoena is a document requiring someone to appear as a witness.

Comparative negligence

Comparative negligence is when each party in a lawsuit absorbs some of the blame and thus the penalty awarded is reduced accordingly.

Vicarious liability

Vicarious liability is a legal responsibility that a person may have for the actions of someone else.

Complaint

Complaint is a document notifying the parties and court in a legal suit what the transactions or occurrences are that will be proved during the proceedings.

Statute

Statute of limitations is the period of time in which a law suit must be started.

Psychosocial & Support Systems

Adaptive and maladaptive family differences

An adaptive family is able to adapt to a crisis, specifically a catastrophic illness, with flexibility, reasonable problem solving, effective communication between the family and the care providers, and the ability to maintain their link to the community.

When a family cannot continue with their own daily functions while meeting the patient's needs, they are a maladaptive family. Maladaptive actions include overindulgence of the patient and/or abandoning other family members, denial of the patient's condition, relying on a single person to provide all assistance to the patient, and failure to seek assistance or accept help from others.

Case Managers must assess the family/support group at the start and throughout the course of an illness by asking probing questions to make sure they understand the scope of the situation. The connection between the family and community resources may determine the level of involvement necessary by the Case Manager to ensure the best result is achieved for the patient.

Patient's belief system

Currently 1 in 10 people living the U.S. are foreign-born; over 40% speak a language other than English at home; and others speak little or no English. This presents Case Managers with clients having diverse cultures, religions and other factors that present barriers or issues in developing treatment plans. Case

Managers must understand the patient's attitudes toward accepting treatment from healthcare providers since their knowledge of illness and health and healing may be based in custom rather than science.

Cultural idiosyncrasies must be taken into account in creating treatment plans that will be followed and thus successful. As examples, Hispanic families usually hold physicians in high regard and may not question their suggestions, however they will turn to the Case Manager with questions. Northern European descendants want to be empowered in their treatment choices. Many African Americans believe healthcare providers are motivated by profit in relation to treatment options. Asian Pacific Americans may concede medical decisions to the family with the eldest son having responsibility to preserve their parent's lives by any means available. Some cultures believe home death is desirable. Through education, Case Managers can become aware of the cultural needs of the community they serve.

DSM-IV guidelines

The Diagnosis and Statistical Manual, DSM-IV, states that an individual must exhibit a significant clinical behavioral or psychological pattern or syndrome associated with one or more of the following conditions:

- illusory distress, such as anxiety or depression
- impaired in an important life functioning activity, such as the ability to work or care for one's self or family
- exhibit a significant increased risk of disability, injury or loss of freedom
- the behavioral pattern is not an expected reaction to a normal

stressful event, such as post-depression following a birth or death.

The most frequent mental disorders that are protected by the Americans with Disabilities Act are contained in Axis I and II of the DSM-IV. Axis I lists mood, anxiety and psychotic disorders, such as panic and posttraumatic stress disorder and bipolar affective disorder. Axis II contains maladaptive personality disorders that can lead to distress of oneself and/or others, such as paranoid or antisocial personality.

Supreme Court's 1999 ADA ruling and the California Fair Employment and Housing Act (FEHA) differences

The Americans with Disabilities Act (ADA) defines a disability as a physical or mental impairment that substantially limits a person's ability in one or more major life activities whether the disability is currently exhibited or historical. However, if medication controls the disability, it cannot be covered by ADA.

The FEHA legislation stated the assessment of the disability must be made without regard to treatment and the limitation needs to only make the major life activity "difficult" for the individual. Case Managers must be familiar with the DSM-IV, Axis V Global Assessment of Functioning (GAF) Scale that provides numerical codes for the levels of an individual's functional capability. ADA protections are not extended to clinical syndromes related to illegal drug use, drinking at work or criminal pathologies such as kleptomania or pyromania.

"Change agent" illness

Any illness that affects an individual's life in physical, social or psychological ways is considered a change agent illness. Change agent illnesses result in loss, anger, fear or anxiety, depression, dependency, loss of self-respect, social status or independence. Catastrophic illnesses, such as closed head or spinal cord injuries are easily recognized as change agents.

Case Managers must recognize that many cases fall into the category of "change agents" due to physical or psychological effects, e.g. a carpenter loses use of a hand or the main breadwinner can no longer function in that capacity. During the intake interview, it is important to document education, support mechanisms, counseling and/or medication that may be needed.

Case follow-up needs to reassess the individual's success at coping with the illness and treatment as, well as the effects on their family and community support group. Addressing the effect on the latter group maintains the patient's support group - the individuals providing social, psychological and even financial support to the patient.

Behavioral health disorders

25% of Americans suffer from behavioral and mental health disorders. Up to 50% of patients with complex medical conditions, especially those with multiple diagnoses will also have mental health or psychiatric problems that will have an influence on their recuperation and healing process. Case Managers are instrumental in identifying the mental or behavioral issues that limit a patient's ability to attend to her healing, including attendance at rehabilitative sessions or follow-up appointments. Case Managers have a responsibility to build their knowledge in psychiatric and behavioral health issues and treatments through attendance at workshops or seminars, reading books and journals, and building relationships with behavioral health professionals including social workers and psychiatrists.

Dealing with end of life issues

Although death is inevitable more than 50% of Americans who are 45 years or older have never discussed end of life (EOL) issues with their families including thoughts about death when someone they loved was terminally ill. Case Managers have the unique position to be able to assist individuals and their families with fact-based information and alleviate their fears.

It is important for Case Managers to know the laws in the state in which they practice. The Patient Self-Determination Act (PSDA) of 1991 requires all Medicare and Medicaid agencies to recognize living wills and powers of attorney for advanced directives in healthcare; however, states have their own definitions and practices regarding guarantees for individual rights to determine treatment. Do not resuscitate (DNR) orders, living wills, healthcare proxies (whishes regarding life-prolonging measures), and other legal documents are areas where Case Managers make an impact on the treatment their clients will receive. These advance directives assist families during crisis situations by allowing discussion and decisions to be made in advance.

Palliative care program

Palliative care program is the process of continual assessment of a patient's needs and their treatment options in accordance with the patient's values and beliefs.

CQI

Continuous quality improvement (CQI) is a key module of total quality management using a meticulous, systematic, organization-wide methodology to achieve ongoing improvement in the quality of healthcare services and operations. CQI looks at both outcomes and processes of care.

Efficacy of care

Efficacy of care is the potential, capacity or capability to achieve the preferred outcome or effect of treatment as previously defined by scientific or research-based findings.

IDS

Integrated delivery system (IDS) refers to a single organization or a group of affiliated organizations providing a wide variety of ambulatory and tertiary care and services.

Axis sections of the DSM-IV classification system

Axis I
Clinical disorders, other disorders that may be a focus of clinical attention. These include disorders usually diagnosed in infancy, childhood or adolescence (excluding mental retardation), delirium, dementia and other cognitive disorders, substance-related, mood, anxiety, and eating or sleep disorders.

Axis II
Personality disorders, mental retardation.

Axis III
General medical conditions (with ICD-9-CM codes)

Axis IV
Psychological and environmental problems, this category includes problems with primary support group or the social environment, educational or occupational problems, housing or economic problems, or problems related to obtaining healthcare or legal services.

<u>Axis V</u>
Global assessment of functioning as defined by the Global Assessment of Function (GAF) scale determined via testing.

DSM

The Diagnostic and Statistical Manual of Mental Disorders (DSM), uses clear English to provide working definitions containing operational criteria for mental disorders. Each disorder is assigned a numerical code that is used by insurance companies for behavioral treatments (such as drug and alcohol treatment or mental retardation).

The manual presents information on each disorder useful to Case Managers including cultural, gender and age-related information, typical clinical treatments, complications and supplies family patterns if the disease has genetic or suspected genetic components. Physicians make the diagnosis, but Case Managers may need to make referrals for testing or observation due to information discovered during client intake or over the course of your relationship with the client.

Physical and mental impairment assessment tools

The Case Manager's assessment must include temporary or permanent functional changes, physiological, psychological, or social problems, possible problems functioning in the community and educational deficits of the patient and family. Although observation is the initial tool used, a variety of test results may be needed to arrive at a diagnostic conclusion including independent medical evaluation, personal interviews and detailed review of all psychiatric records.

The Minn. Multiphasic Personality Inventory, Ranchos Los Amigos Levels of Cognitive Functions and Glasgow Coma Scale are assessment tools used frequently in initial and continued assessment of a patient. The results of the tests assist the Case Manager in designing the individualized plan for placement of the patient and the level of services needed. Stroke, brain trauma and spinal cord injuries/lesions patients require vastly different treatment plans and equipment depending on the location and extent of the problem. Family members may not have formal testing, but their level of cognition must be noted in the case file in order to create an individualized plan for the patient.

Ranchos Los Amigos Levels

Ranchos Los Amigos Levels of Cognitive Functioning are as follows:
- I = No response: Totally unresponsive to all stimuli
- II = Generalized response: Inconsistent or non-purposeful reactions; delayed reaction to deep pain stimuli
- III = Localized response: Specific but inconsistent reactions; reaction in a manner not related to the stimuli
- IV = Confused/agitated: Short attention span, confusion, excited behavior, impaired speech, tires easily, no cooperation in his treatment plan
- V = Confused/inappropriate: Patient is alert and responsive to simple commands and familiar people, needs structure, may wander and may have memory impairment
- VI = Confused appropriate: Patient has goal-directed behavior but needs structure, aware of environment, has the ability to

learn but needs frequent repetition

- VII = Automatic/appropriate: Follows a daily routine but cannot deal with unexpected situations, vague understanding of his condition but no real cognition of the details or the future
- VIII = Purposeful/appropriate: Alert and oriented, functioning within confines of the current injury, understands a skill once learned without supervision, able to function in society unless an unexpected or stressful situation occurs

HIV Prevention Case Management

Prevention case management (PCM) links clients with the services they need, providing coordination and brokerage of services beyond what the client might be able to obtain without the benefit of a Case Manager. For persons living with HIV, coordination needs to exist between health care, psychiatric, psychosocial, and other community support services.

For clients with HIV, there needs to be identification of risk behaviors and development of a prevention plan that outlines specific behavioral objectives.

Part of the medical and psychosocial services includes STD evaluation and treatment and substance abuse treatment. The goal of HIV primary prevention is reduction of the transmission and acquisition of HIV infection. The goal of HIV secondary prevention is to prevent a person with HIV from becoming ill or dying as a result of HIV-related illness. HIV prevention case management requires community understanding and support. It is important to understand the norms, values and traditions sanctioned by the community leaders and accepted by the population in order to succeed in PCM. In other words, the Case Manager must have cultural competence.

CDC for prevention case management of HIV/AIDS

Clear procedure and protocol manuals must list the standards of care, the quality assurance procedures, and be available to all staff. Client feedback should be sought in assessing the quality of the services provided. The following should be included in quality assurance assessments:

- Descriptions of communication tools (intake and follow up forms, partner notification, and risk-reduction counseling)
- Description of training provided to supervisors and staff along with job descriptions
- Staff performance reviews
- Chart reviews including initial assessment, prevention plan, and progress notes on clients
- Presentation of cases by case managers to peers and supervisors which include intervention strategy discussions
- Review by peers of the quality of services being provided
- Feedback from clients including satisfaction, concerns and their ideas for improvements
- Reviews and evaluations from outside professionals which verify that the services being promoted are being delivered

Healthcare Management & Delivery

Identifying potential case management patients

The five methods of identifying potential case management patients are:

1) Payers will often identify catastrophic diagnosis cases where complex, multiple care providers and services will be costly for both the patient and payer. These include HIV/AIDS, head injuries, neurological and back surgery, bone marrow transplants, etc.
2) High risk diagnoses may lead to high-cost services. These include pregnancy induced hypertension, new onset seizure disorder, malignant cardiac arrhythmia, etc.
3) Procedures that are associated with catastrophic diseases are called sentinel procedures. Case Managers should review scheduling of these procedures. Some examples are major organ biopsies, arteriovenous shunt placement, and exploratory laparotomy
4) Any time an admitting diagnoses rises above the predetermined cost, the Case Manager should review the file. This is termed high cost case selection resulting from misleading or masked admitting diagnosis or unforeseen complications
5) Passive case acquisitions are received from requests for services from community members. The term "passive" refers to the fact that the Case

Manager did not solicit the case and had no involvement in case selection. Direct case referral comes from established criteria and rules for case referrals

Hospital length of stay

Hospital length of stay as defined by NMHPA begins at the time of the newborn's delivery, or the last delivery time in the event of multiple births, when the birth occurs at a hospital. If the delivery occurs outside the hospital, length of stay begins at the time the mother or newborn is admitted to the hospital in connection with the childbirth. Only the physician can determine that the admittance is "in connection with childbirth."

Ancillary services

Ancillary services are those diagnostic and therapeutic services needed by a patient other than nursing or medicine. These include respiratory, laboratory, radiology, nutrition, physical and occupational therapy and pastoral services.

Intervention

It is the planned strategies and activities that address a maladaptive behavior or state of being and assist growth and change. Another term for intervention is treatment when used to describe medical treatment strategies. Examples of intervention are advocacy, psychotherapy or speech language therapy.

HIPAA's main objectives

HIPAA is the Health Insurance Portability and Accountability Act of 1996 and is recognized as one of the most important legislative acts impacting healthcare since the Medicare programs of 1965.

- 48 -

Title I guarantees health insurance access, portability and renewal when a person needs to change insurance plans; eliminates some preexisting condition clauses and does not allow for discrimination based on health status.

Title II establishes the majority of the rules and requirements the healthcare industry must follow under HIPAA addressing the integrity of health coverage by creating fraud and abuse controls, demanding adherence to Administrative Simplification (AS) standards which reduces paperwork, addressing medical liability reform and guaranteeing the security and privacy of health information.

Title III allows medical savings accounts and tax deductions for insurance premiums of the self-employed.

Title IV gives the enforcement of the HIPAA provisions to the Office of Civil Rights.

Title V creates revenue offset provisions.

HIPAA Title II AS provisions

Standardizing patient health information and financial data and use of Electronic Data Interchange (EDI) transactions reduces both transaction time and administrative costs. Medical providers, insurers, payers and to a small extent employers submit enrollment forms and claims electronically and receive payments in the same manner. Security standards protect the confidentiality and integrity of all information using unique identifiers for individuals, employers, health plans and healthcare providers.

Case Managers must comply with the confidentiality standards by protecting the identity of their clients, their families and the service providers. HIPAA

compliance is required in use of fax, phone, and Internet communications.

"Preexisting condition"

Any diagnosed and treated medical condition within six (6) months before the enrollment date of a health insurance policy qualifies as a preexisting condition and can be excluded from medical coverage under a new policy.

To exclude a health issue from insurance coverage, the preexisting condition must have been diagnosed and either treated or have recommended treatment within 6 months prior to the enrollment date. Exclusion date begins at the start of the enrollment wait period if one applies. Exclusion of the condition cannot last more than 12 months (18 months for late enrollees) from the date of enrollment.

The exclusion is reduced by the number of days of the individual's prior creditable coverage (without more than 63 days break in coverage). The following cannot be considered preexisting conditions: pregnancy, newborn or adopted children under 18, children placed for adoption who have been covered under the health plan for at least 30 days.

State changes to HIPAA

States rights take precedence over HIPAA if the state's laws are stricter in protecting medical records privacy. There are only several areas where states may legislate stricter requirements on health insurance providers. It is important to check with the State Insurance Commissioner's Office to obtain their modifications.
- States may shorten the preexisting condition 6 month timeframe
- Shorten the maximum preexisting condition time period (12 or 18 months)

- 49 -

- Increase the insurance break period to more than 63 days
- Increase the 30 day enrollment period for newborns and adopted children
- Add to the health conditions which cannot be subjected to preexisting conditions exclusions
- Require additional special enrollment periods
- Reduce the HMO affiliation period to less than 2 months (3 months for late enrollees)

Health insurance waiting period

Insurance plans or issuers can require a waiting period before the start of coverage. Preexisting conditions waiting period begins when the policy waiting period begins, not the first day of insurance coverage.

Creditable coverage

Creditable coverage references the time during which a person is covered by health insurance, including COBRA continuation coverage.

Break in coverage

A significant break in coverage is a span of 63 days or more without health insurance. To calculate creditable coverage, credit is granted to coverage without any break in that coverage of 63 days or more. Coverage that ended more than 63 days from the new enrollment will not be credited against a preexisting condition. A certificate of coverage must be issued by group health plans and health insurance issuers.

Levels of healthcare

Acute care is short term medical treatment, usually in a hospital, for episodic illness or injury.

Long-term care applies to major trauma patients or those with chronic and multiple medical, mental and social problems who cannot take care of themselves.

Custodial care is mainly for the purpose of assisting clients with their home personal care and does not necessarily require the provider to have specialized skills or training.

Intermediate care applies to patients requiring more than custodial care and might require nursing supervision. Unless true skilled care is required, insurance companies group intermediate and custodial care under the same benefit guidelines.

Skilled nursing and sub-acute care describe a patient who needs to be medically stable and the level of care is sub-acute rather than acute. Treatments in this level include frequent or complex wound care, rehabilitation, complex intravenous therapy, and combination therapies. Patients are usually in an extended care facility (ECF) such as a nursing home or a skilled nursing facility.

Transitional hospital

Transitional hospitals are acute care facilities for patients that are medically stable and whose rehabilitation plan is too complex for an extended care facility (ECF). Transitional hospitals that specialize in medically complex care do so at a lower cost than a traditional hospital because of their specialization. Some transitional hospitals supply only basic patient care, also at a lower cost than a traditional hospital. Examples of transitional hospitals are: burn or extensive could care; hemodialysis; hospice; infectious disease management; Intravenous (IV) medication therapies; neurobehavioral rehabilitation; pain control therapies; rehabilitation; total parenteral nutrition; and ventilator care/weaning from ventilators.

Practicality of including home care treatment assessment

Home care is the fastest growing component of healthcare due to viability of even complex care being handled in the home (e.g. ventilators, total parenteral nutrition or infusion care). The Case Manager must look at the medical, financial and social situation of the patient to determine if home care is a viable option.

Managed care has spearheaded the home care alternative and Medicare has allowed the care with contracts with health maintenance organizations (HMOs). The Case Manager must review the patient's insurance coverage benefits for the necessary treatments before recommending home care versus facility care. Traditionally the following criteria must be met for home health visits:
- the patient is confined to their home or have great difficulty going to an outpatient facility
- the care requires intermittent skilled nursing services and may include physical, occupational and speech therapies
- the patient's care plan is reasonable and medically necessary and is overseen by a physician who reviews the care plan at least every 60 days
- the home healthcare agency is Medicare-certified meeting the strictest federal standards

Hospice

Hospice is a healthcare program that provides support and comfort to patients and the families dealing with the final stages of terminal illness. The goal is to provide care at home, although specialized hospice facilities exist in many locations. Medicare covers hospice care if:
- a physician certifies the patient is terminally ill
- the patient or family requests hospice assistance
- the provider is Medicare-certified

The physician's hospice referral can be made from either a home or hospital setting. To receive hospice care coverage, a patient must waive standard Medicare benefits for the illness/condition causing the hospice referral, however, care for other conditions unrelated to the hospice referral condition are covered by standard Medicare benefits. Medicare Part A pays for two 90-day and one 30 day benefit periods (210 days out of 7 months) but extensions can be obtained for long duration terminal illnesses.

Types of transportation

A Case Manager can arrange transportation for patients who are so infirm that assistance is required to/from healthcare facilities (from one hospital to another) due to medical necessity. Coverage by health plans is not usually available from a healthcare facility to the patient's home.

Wheelchair vans or ambulette services may be used for stable patients or those with their own oxygen who do not need it regulated by a professional. Wheelchair van transportation is rarely a covered benefit. Ground transportation ambulances are generally two types:
1) Basic life support (BLS) which includes limited monitoring by a BLS paramedic
2) Advanced life support (ALS) which includes an ALS paramedic, cardiac monitoring and a drug box. This is the most common

transportation between acute
care and rehabilitation hospitals

Air ambulances provide advanced cardiac life support (ACLS) personnel, cardiac monitoring and a medication box along with a registered nurse. Unless arranged by a Case Manager, air transportation is usually not covered by health plans; exceptions may be transportation from an inaccessible region (e.g. mountaintop) or speeding to a hospital for an approved organ transplant.

Durable medical equipment

Durable medical equipment must be appropriate for use in the home, have a medical/therapeutic purpose, withstand repeated use, allow sterilization or disinfection between uses, and not be useful in the absence of illness or injury. Durable medical equipment may be:
- a basic mobility device such as a walker or crutches
- an assistive device for activities of daily living such as bathroom equipment, incontinence, wound care or feeding/kitchen aids
- extensive mobility equipment such as a wheelchair, motorized scooter or hospital bed
- advanced high-tech equipment such as oxygen, ventilator, infusion pump or sleep monitor

Case Managers must understand the equipment handled by various vendors and establish a relationship with the vendors in order to offer the patient a choice of vendors and monitor/report on the success of the patient. The vendor assists the Case Manger by procuring equipment at the appropriate time, setting up the equipment, instructing the patient and their caregivers on the use of the equipment, handling repairs/replacement of equipment, and completing insurance paperwork.

Monitoring patients use
The Case Manager has the responsibility to monitor a patient's use of durable medical equipment, amend their individualized treatment plan as changes in the need for use of the equipment occur and report on the overall relationship with the vendor. Vendors should assist or at least supply criteria for the proposed equipment. In ordering and placing equipment in the home, the Case Manager must be aware of the physical layout of the house so that equipment that cannot be operated in the space available will not be ordered. The physical dimensions of the patient must be taken into account as well as changes that will occur over the duration of the equipment use (e.g. children's growth, reduction in weight, small adults needing child-size equipment).

The Case Manager must determine if the patient is using the equipment correctly or not at all, removing unused equipment. Progressive disabilities need close monitoring to adjust equipment in accordance with the advance of the disease. For long term disabilities, it may be more economical to purchase versus rent equipment. Case Managers can work with vendors to arrange for rental fees to be applied to purchases, documenting the information for presentation to the insurance provider.

Orthosis and prosthesis

An orthosis is a device that assists the body in restoring a function. It can be a sling, brace, or splint that is added to a person's body to achieve one of the following: support, posture, immobilization, correct deformities, assist weak muscles, restore muscle function, and/or modify muscle tone. An orthosis can be simple, made of cotton (sling) or plastic, or a complex electromechanical appliance containing cantilevered joints or servomotors.

Prosthesis is a device that replaces all or part of a missing body part or replaces a body part that is no longer functioning. Prosthesis vary and are individualized for looks and functionality. Prosthesis include lens replacement following cataract surgery, a hip replacement, artificial arms and legs, breast implants following mastectomy, or a wig due to chemotherapy.

Fitting a transtibial prosthesis

The Case Manager needs to understand the stages of prosthesis creation by the trained and certified professionals they recommend. There are six (6) steps in fitting a transtibial (below the knee) prosthesis:

1) Fitting requires making a cast of the stump, taking care to push in on the soft prominences and avoiding the bony ones
2) The prosthetist makes a model marking the bony prominences so that weight will be transferred to the soft tissue areas around the distal end
3) The interface is the part of the prosthesis that touches the residual limb, holding and stabilizing the prosthesis, bearing the body weight, and protecting the residual limb from damage due to friction and weight bearing. First a clear plastic interface is made
4) This allows alignment of the prosthesis so that measurements and adjustments are easily made. During the alignment phase, adjustments to the moving parts of the prosthesis are also done
5) The definitive prosthesis is made once the fitting of the interface and alignments are complete. As a rule, the average amputee is fully functional within a year of his amputation
6) Finally repair and replacement and adjustment and maintenance are the final steps in prosthesis' life

Assistive device characteristics

Assistive or adaptive devices are products that allow an individual to be more independent in performing activities when they have impaired abilities or functional limitations. The device may be used on a temporary basis during treatment or they may be a long term solution following reasonable effort to learn the task. The assessment for use of an assistive device is similar to the overview needed for use of durable medical equipment.

Assistive devices include the following categories: visual aids (glasses, audio books); hears aids; speaking/communicating devices (text-to-voice synthesizer); orientation to time/place/person (memory books, clocks); ambulation/location (cane, walker, wheelchair); eating (nonskid mat for plates, rocker knife); dressing (button hook); toileting (toilet seat with rails, bedside commode); shower/tub (grab bars, tub chair, hand-held nozzle); transfer (gait belt, hydraulic lifts for bed/chair/stairs); and recreation (large print books, video games, fishing pole harness).

The patient and caregivers need to be involved in the selection of the device and understand its use. Documentation for the need of the device must be provided by the Case Manager for the insurance provider to cover the costs.

Joint Commission on Accreditation of Healthcare Organizations

Established in 1951, the Joint Commission is an independent, nonprofit organization whose purpose is to improve the quality of care provided patients. Organizations/facilities attaining accreditation meet established, quality performance standards allowing them to waive specific licensure requirements and meet certain Medicare certification requirements.

Rehabilitation Accreditation Commission

Established in 1966, CARF establishes standards of quality for organizations providing rehabilitation services. CARF believes all people have the right to be treated with respect and dignity, have access to needed services to achieve optimal outcomes, and should be empowered to make informed choices. Organizations with CARF accreditation actively involve consumers in the selection and planning of services that are state-of-the-art and they focus on assisting each patient in achieving their chosen outcomes.

Board Certifications

There are 24 specialty boards recognized by the American Board of Medical Specialties and the American Medical Association which certify that physicians have met approved education and knowledge-retention requirements. Certifications are issued for specific periods of time requiring practitioners to continue their education and re-certify.

Augmentative communication device

An AAC, augmentative and alternative communication device is used to assist or augment a person in communicating. The device may be as simple as a picture board containing items or activities that a person can point to or as complex as a computerized system allowing input from a keyboard, head stick or eye gaze switch which produces synthesized speech.

Chinwand or chinstick

Chinwand or chinstick is a device that is mounted to a headpiece and extends from the center of the mandible allowing a person with good head mobility, but poor upper body strength, to make selections on an input device (AAC). A similar device extending from the forehead is called a headwand or headstick.

Dial scan

Dial scan is a device that looks like a clock with one hand. The single hand points to pictures or symbols activating switch which operates the item.

CMG

Case mix group is a patient classification system based on diagnoses used to describe the types of patients treated at a hospital.

Comorbidity

Comorbidity is the term that describes a condition where there is a primary condition plus many other conditions affecting an individual. An auto injury patient may be treated for a heart attack while also having broken bones or diabetes. In psychiatry there may be an Axis I major depressive disorder while also being an Axis II personality disorder. There is as yet no standard, accepted "test" to determine the primary, secondary, tertiary, etc. order of the diseases.

MDS

Minimum data set is an assessment tool used by skilled nursing facilities to determine the clinical needs of residents placing them in a Resource Utilization Group (RUG). The RUG determines the reimbursement rate the skilled nursing facility receives from Medicare. The RUG has 7 major categories and 44 minor categories based on the MDS assessment.

Patient's bill of rights

The Patient's Bill of Rights was first adopted in 1973 by the American Hospital Association then revised in October 1992. Each facility produces their Patient Bill of Rights incorporating state laws and hospital policies. It provides empowerment to the patient for making informed decisions about their medical care.

It encourages patients to create an advance directive, such as a living will, healthcare proxy or durable power of attorney, so that if they are incapacitated their treatment wishes will be honored.

The Bill of Rights states the rights the patient has for privacy and their ability to review their medical records and have information explained in common, understandable language. Hospitals must reveal their relationship with other businesses or educational institutions that could affect the care the patient will receive. The Bill of Rights also includes information on how to resolve disputes or grievances. Patients are also made aware of their role in maintaining their continued health and recovery.

HIV/AIDS patient challenges

AIDS has become the largest pandemic in history, affecting 800,000-900,000 people in the U.S. and approximately 40,000 new cases annually. It is a disease of the immune system that allows other diseases to invade the body. The spread of AIDS is due to risky behavior (any sexual behavior and drug/needle sharing), drug resistance, noncompliance, and the denial of AIDS. AIDS is a quick multiplier turning over every 30 minutes.

40% of HIV/AIDS patients also have hepatitis C which also requires toxic and rigid drug treatment. Because AIDS compromises the immune system, complications and coexisting conditions occur. AIDS clients require long-term care case management, and increased awareness of confidentiality, social stigmatization, prejudice, and manipulation of benefits.

Barriers and roadblocks are often encountered in trying to coordinate treatments and resources for AIDS patients. Due to confidentiality, benefits may be denied based on a diagnostic code and interference by the Case Manager can resolve the issues. Case Managers need to empower AIDS clients to take an active role in the management of their treatment. The patient is the first to recognize changes and communication with their case manager allows realignment of the treatment plan.

AIDS cases

It is important for Case Mangers to examine their beliefs and feelings about death before handling AIDS cases. It is important not to pre-judge the patient based on their AIDS diagnosis.

Understanding AIDS and the diseases associated with AIDS is important in providing services to the patient. Knowing community resources and educational sources including Internet sites are important aspects of managing

AIDS cases and assisting the patient in self-management of their treatment.

Understanding your feelings about death will enable the Case Manager to cope with the loss of an AIDS patient. The Case Manager needs to be prepared to cope with the inevitable death of the patient, someone who shared intimate details of their life or their thoughts about suicide due to the physical degradation they will suffer. Conversely, the Case Manager may need to deal with someone in denial of their demise. It is important for the Case Manager to avoid painting a positive picture of the outcome of the treatment plan, a view contrary to the Case Manager's usual patient interaction. The Case Manager may need to identify their own support mechanism while handling AIDS cases.

Longer life for HIV/'AIDS clients

The title Case Manager implies "management" not "monitoring." In handling AIDS cases, it is important for Case Managers to inquire about new therapies and drug interactions and obtain research information about the disease. Advances in antiretroviral drug and protease inhibitor combinations (triple cocktails), along with an understanding of the effects of nutrition and supplements, has moved HIV infections into chronic disease, long-term care. Case Managers can stress wellness and prevention strategies in the treatment plans as well as including return-to-work scenarios.

The key to surviving with HIV is early diagnosis and starting therapy, use of viral load indicators and CD4+ T-cell counts, aggressive treatments using a minimum of 3 drugs, recognition and identification of opportunistic infections and protein-calorie malnutrition, restoration of the immune system,

understanding mind-body connection, and empowering the HIV-infected person to assume self-management.

Assisting the individual in understanding the importance of maintaining body weight (adds 10 years) is another key factor in stopping HIV from advancing to AIDS. The disease consumes calories. A 10% reduction of body weight reduces life expectancy and over 30% of patients die from "wasting syndrome."

Triple cocktails for AIDS patients

Triple cocktails are combinations of antiretroviral drugs that reduce HIV virus levels. Reduction of the virus to below detection level reduces the incidence of opportunistic diseases and slows other signs of the diseases progression. Drug treatments are expensive ($12,000-$15,000/year) and must be ingested in a specific sequence within a specific time period.

The administration of the drugs presents a challenge to patients and care givers, the drugs have debilitating side effects and effect different patients in different ways, and are only effective in 30% of patients, in part due to the difficulty in administering the drugs. Case Managers need to be aware of toxicity and resistance issues with HIV patients. The drugs compete with one another causing reactions and they also interact with foods to cause side effects. Protease inhibitors can cause metabolic upheaval such as maldistribution of body fat resulting in a disproportional look.

HIV drugs can cause adverse interactions in combination with over-the-counter and certain prescription drugs. Case Managers need to be aware of harmful drug interactions. Assisting patients in researching and obtaining drugs through free distribution programs, direct from

- 56 -

manufacturers or becoming part of research studies is an important role for Case Managers.

Disease management

Case Management focuses on an individual; disease management, or condition management, focuses on populations with widespread, often chronic, diseases with varying care practices. Non-disease conditions, such as pregnancy or cessation of smoking, are also candidates for disease/condition management. Participants are identified via claims review, new member health assessments or provider referrals.

Disease management allows knowledge to be transferred among the population and care providers. Case Managers may be assigned responsibility to communicate with participants in disease/condition management programs sending out information or informing participants of educational opportunities. Just as in case management, disease management resources should be documented and the savings of using sound management processes should be calculated and reported.

Health policy reimbursement

Private health insurance pays the cost of Long Term Care (LTC) when medically necessary. If the limit of private insurance is reached or care is considered custodial, Medicaid pays the cost. Medicare pays 100% of the first 20 days in a skilled nursing facility (SNF) and then 80% up to a total of 100 inpatient days if there is a medical necessity.

Skilled nursing and sub-acute care placements require the Case Manager to understand specific policy benefits and whether or not the insurer will coordinate payment with Medicare. The

20% not covered by Medicare may be the patient's liability. Most insurers make very little distinction between intermediate and custodial care in distributing benefits. Inpatient rehabilitation has specific qualifiers for private policies which may or may not be the same as the Medicare admission criteria.

Inpatient rehabilitation Medicare admission criteria

Inpatient rehabilitation is an intense program and some patients may go from acute care to a sub-acute or SNF setting first. To qualify under Medicare, the patient must meet the four main admittance criteria:

1) Admitting diagnosis includes one of the following: amputation; arthritis; cardiac, orthopedic or pulmonary conditions; cerebral vascular, congenital, musculoskeletal, or neurological disorders; chronic pain; diabetes mellitus; fracture; head trauma/brain injury; multiple trauma; or spinal cord injury
2) Admission must be for a recent functional loss that the patient was able to carry out prior to the injury or illness
3) The diagnosis by the physician must have an expectation for significant improvement in the functional deficit in a reasonable amount of time
4) If the patient had already been in a rehabilitative program for the problem, their condition must have changed such that progress is now possible

Medicare eligibility

Medicare is the nation's largest health insurance program covering over 40 million Americans. Medicare covers people:

- 65 years old and receiving or are eligible for benefits through the Social Security or Railroad Retirement systems or the patient's spouse has Medicare-covered government employment.
- Disabled people are entitle to Medicare once they are on Social Security disability benefits for 24 months, and then complete the five-month waiting period, e.g. a total of 29 months.
- Diagnosed with permanent kidney failure or end-stage renal disease (ESRD) meaning they are on dialysis or require a transplant
- Social Security or Railroad retirement benefits must also be met and they have a 3 month waiting period before benefits begin
- Benefits end 3 months following the end of dialysis or 36 months following a transplant. Illness other than ESRD is not covered for people who do not meet regular Medicare eligibility
- If a patient is already enrolled in a Medicare Managed Care Plan/Health Maintenance Organization (HMO), the plan will cover their kidney failure treatments, otherwise, once diagnosed they cannot join a plan

Graph of Medicare Payments

Hospital Treatment
- In-hospital days Medicare pays/Patient pays
- 1st to 60th 100% of allowable charges minus deductible
- Part A deductible = $764.00
- 61st to 90th
- 100% of allowable charges minus Part A coinsurance

- Part A coinsurance = $191.00*
- 91st to 151st
- 100% of allowable charges minus Part A coinsurance
- Part A coinsurance = $382.00*

Medigap and Medicare Select

Patients are responsible for Medicare's coinsurance, deductible fees and many medical services not covered, (e.g. prescriptions).

Medigap is private insurance which helps pay these "gaps." Medigap's open enrollment period is 6 months from the date of enrollment in Medicare Part B and age 65 or older. Open enrollment means the patient cannot be turned down or charged higher premiums due to poor health, factors that limit Medigap options after the open enrollment period.

Another type of supplemental health insurance is Medicare Select. Medicare Select is a health maintenance organization-type policy that specifies the hospitals, and in some cases providers a patient must use, unless there is an emergency. Due to the provider restrictions, Medicare Select usually offers more reasonable premiums than Medigap policies.

Insurance other than Medicare

Many people have both Medicare and private health insurance coverage. The private policy will pay first when:
- the individual is 65 or older
- the patient or their spouse is working at an employer with 20 or more employees with group health insurance based on the employment
- the individual is under 65 and disabled
- the individual or family member carrying the insurance works for a

company with 100 or more employees
- the individual has Medicare based on kidney failure
- Worker's Compensation, federal black lung program, no-fault insurance, or any liability insurance is covering the illness or injury

Balanced Budget Act of 1997

The Balanced Budget Act of 1997 provided coverage of preventive care recognizing it as cost-effective. Procedures covered include:

1) one influenza vaccination per year and one pneumococcal vaccine per lifetime
2) one mammogram for women over 40 with no Part B deductible
3) one PAP smear and one pelvic exam every 3 years, unless the woman is at high risk and the Part B deductible waived and one colorectal cancer screening each year for people over 50
4) diabetic education and glucose test strips to achieve outpatient self-management
5) osteoporosis bone mass tests for people who are clinical at risk for osteoporosis
6) yearly prostate cancer screening for men over 50

Categorically needy and the needy eligibility groups for Medicaid coverage

Title XIX of the Social Security Act established Medicaid as a national insurance program for the poor and categorically or medically needy. States set the eligibility requirements using the minimum standards set by CMS.

Categorically needy are families and certain children who qualify for public assistance, (e.g. Aid to Families with Dependent Children (AFDC) or Supplemental Security Income (SSI), and include the aged, blind and physically disabled adults and children).

Medically needy eligible individuals or families with sufficient earnings to meet their basic needs but do not have the resources to pay healthcare bills. Low income is not the only criteria for Medicaid eligibility; assets and other resources are considered. Medically needy often qualify for coverage due to excessive medical expenses and the benefits may be confined to that specific illness only, e.g. tuberculosis (TB).

Medicaid categorically needy assistance groups

The following are examples of Medicaid categorically needy assistance groups:
- AFDC recipients
- SSI recipients or any of the following who as of 1/1/72 were in a State's Medicaid plan: aged, blind and disabled individuals
- Infants born to Medicaid-eligible women and the children remain in the program for the next 12 months plus 60 days after the end of the pregnancy as long as the mother remains eligible for the program
- Children under age 6 and pregnant women who meet the state's AFDC financial requirements or the SSI program for pregnant women. Also, any family whose income is at or below 133% of the federal poverty level (FPL), or the minimum mandatory income level for pregnant women and infants in their state. Pregnant women remain eligible for Medicaid through the end of the calendar month that falls 60 days following

the end of the pregnancy, even if their income status changes

- Families who receive adoption assistance and foster care under Title IV-E of the Social Security Act.

Medicate and matching federal funds

Matching federal funds under Medicaid are provided to states who apply more liberal guidelines for categorically need families. These optional groups are:

- Infants up to age 1 and pregnant women whose income is below 185% of the federal poverty level (or the percentage set by the state) and not covered under the mandatory rules
- Some aged, blind or disabled adults whose income is above the mandatory coverage limit but below the federal poverty level
- Children under 21 who meet AFDC income and resource requirements but otherwise are not eligible for AFDC
- Institutionalized individuals with income and resources below specified limits
- Individuals receiving care via home and community-based services but would be eligible if institutionalized
- Beneficiaries of state supplementary payments
- TB-infected individuals who meet the financial eligibility for Medicaid at the SSI level for their TB-related ambulatory services and TB drugs only

Medicaid program basic tenants

Medicaid is a national insurance program, created by Title XIX of the Social Security Act, for the poor and "needy" in all states and territories. There are no "out of pocket" medical expenses for persons covered by Medicaid. Medicaid is funded by federal and state governments and usually administered by state welfare or health departments. Although coverage varies from state to state/territory, it must always cover:

- Inpatient hospital care and outpatient services
- Physicians' services; 3) skilled nursing homes for adults
- Laboratory and x-ray services
- Family planning services; NS
- Preventative and periodic screening, diagnosis and treatment for children under age 21

Spousal Impoverishment

The Medicaid Catastrophic Coverage Act (MCCA) allows Medicaid coverage for an individual in an institution if income levels are met after deductions for minimum monthly spousal community living expenses are taken into account.

The patient must have an expected stay in a nursing home or medical facility for at least 30 days. To determine how much of the income/assets will be used to support the spouse in the medical facility, the spousal resource amount (SRA) is calculated by taking the combined spousal assets, minus the house, car, household goods, and burial costs and dividing by two: SRA = ½ x (combined assets) – (house, car, etc.).

The SRA is compared to the state's minimum resource standard ($76,740 in 1996). If it is more, The SRA is deducted from the minimum standard with that remainder applied to the costs of the spouse's expenses in the medical facility. The spouse remaining in the community has the remainder, the spouse protected resource amount (PRA).

Spouse Medicaid Catastrophic Coverage

Once an individual in a medical/nursing facility is determined to be eligible for Medicaid, the post-eligibility process is used to determine how much the spouse in the medical facility must contribute toward the cost of their care. Take the total income of the spouse residing in the facility and deduct in the following order:

- $30/month for personal allowance
- The community spouse's monthly income allowance (in 1996 between $1,295 and $1,918.50)
- A family monthly income allowance
- An amount for the medical expenses of the spouse in the medical facility
- The total deductions subtracted from the income of the spouse in the medical facility equals the amount that individual must contribute toward their cost of care

Ramifications of transferring assets

When state/federal funding is requested to assist in paying for long-term care facility, receiving home, or community-based waiver services, the financial records of the individual will be examined by the state. Both real assets and income are taken into account, and any transfers for less than their fair market value will be questioned.

The state "looks back" 36 months before the date the individual enters the facility or the date Medicaid is applied for. The look back can extend 60 months. Any transfer of assets for less than fair market value is subject to a penalty period, a period of time that a state will withhold payment for a nursing facility or other long-term care services.

The penalty period is calculated by dividing the true worth of the asset by the average cost of the facility in that state. The following are the exceptions to imposing a penalty period:

- when the transfer was done to benefit a spouse
- to certain disabled individuals or a trust for the individual
- when the transfer was for a reason other than Medicaid qualification
- when undue hardship would result from the penalty

Treatment of trusts in regards to Medicaid eligibility

A trust is property held by a person or trust company (the trustee) for the benefit of another (the beneficiary). The grantor is the person or entity that establishes the trust and puts in the assets. Revocable trusts allow the terms or beneficiaries to be changed and irrevocable trusts do not allow any changes in the terms or beneficiaries.

Trust payments or amounts that could be paid to the individual in a medical/nursing facility are also treated as available resources in calculating Medicaid eligibility. Assets that cannot be paid or benefit the individual, but were transferred to the trust at less than market value to meet Medicaid eligibility, are subject to a penalty period during look back.

The following trust situations cannot be counted as available resources:

- Set up by a parent, grandparent, guardian or court for a disabled individual under 65 using the individual's own funds
- Set up by a disabled individual, parent, grandparent, guardian or court for a disabled individual, using the person's own revenues

or pooled funds, managed by a nonprofit organization and used for the sole benefit of each person included in the trust
- Containing pension, Social Security and other income of the individual, in states where individuals are eligible for institutional care under a special income level, but the trust does not cover the care for the medically needy
- When the state determines that counting the trust would cause under hardship

SSI

SSI, Supplemental Security Income, is a federal program run by the Social Security Administration, but using general tax funds, to provide supplemental income to the aged, or any age person who is blind or disabled. To receive SSI you do not need to be receiving Social Security benefits, but must have very limited income and personal property. Limited income and property is defined as less than $2000 for an individual or $3000 for a couple.

Monthly income is dependent on where the individual lives and the following guidelines:
- Not working and monthly income of $490/individual or $725/couple or working income of $1250/individual or $1495/couple

The following assets are not taken into consideration:
- Individual's home
- Household goods up to $2000
- Wedding rings
- Car
- Trade or business property used for self-support

- Value of burial plot
- Up to $1500 for burial expense
- Cash value of life insurance if less than $1500

SSI for disabled individuals
SSI Eligibility under disability means any individual, regardless of age, who cannot engage in substantial gainful employment, cannot work due to a medically diagnosed physical or mental impairment, or whose medical impairment will result in death or in a disability lasting 12 months or more.

SSI payments are independent of any Social Security benefits. Most SSI recipients also receive medical care through the Medicaid program. The basic amount of SSI payments is $470 for one person or $705 for couples. Some states supplement SSI and if there are other sources of income, SSI checks may be less than the basic amount.

SCHIP program

SCHIP is the State Children's Health Insurance Program. It was established in 1997 by the federal government to providing matching funds to states for health insurance coverage for children.

States set their eligibility following federal guidelines. Recipients must have low income, not be eligible for Medicaid and have no health insurance coverage. SCHIP covers, at a minimum, inpatient and outpatient hospital services; doctors' surgical and medical services, laboratory and x-ray services, and well-baby/child care, including immunizations.

OASDI

OASDI is the Old-Age, Survivors' and Disability Insurance program which is the centerpiece of the Social Security Act. It provides hospital insurance to the elderly and supplementary medical insurance for other medical costs.

Health insurance coverage types

Indemnity health insurance plan is a legal entity, licensed by the state insurance department, providing reimbursement for healthcare claims.

Managed indemnity companies are those who have adopted cost-saving approaches to healthcare coverage.

Self-insured is an alternative option adopted by many companies where all or part of the coverage risk, up to a threshold amount, is assumed by the employer rather than an insurance company.

For costs incurred over the individual employee's threshold amount, the employer purchases a re-insurance, or a stop-loss, policy which then pays the remainder of a claim.

Automobile insurance provides coverage for medical expenses and lost wages when the car owner/policy holder has an accident. They must also be aware that when auto insurance maximums are reached, the healthcare plan may be used to complete treatment. Many auto accidents go to court and the Case Manager records may be subpoenaed.

Managed Care is a cost-containment healthcare system overseen by an organization other than the physician or patient. Managed care encompasses:
- HMOs (health maintenance organizations)
- PPOs (preferred provider organizations)
- EPOs (exclusive provider organizations)
- POS (point of service) plans

TPA relationship to self-insurance health plans

A TPA (Third Party Administrator) performs administrative functions for self-insured employers. The services include, but are not limited to, performing claims review and payment, maintaining records, reporting on utilization, providing case management, and overseeing the provider network.

Using a TPA usually provides significant costs savings over the company administering its self-insurance internally. A TPA decreases the start up time by providing computerization of the healthcare plan and administrative expertise. A TPA eliminates the expense of hiring employees to oversee the insurance program.

TPA fees cover the computer costs involved in maintaining the self-insurance and meeting all HIPAA requirements. A TPA also provides objectivity in claims review as they are not direct employees of the company. Furthermore, a TPA provides consulting services to the company on state and federal regulations regarding insurance plans since self-insurance avoids minimum benefits required by state and federal regulations.

HMOs types

Staff model is comprised of physicians who work only for, and are paid by, the HMO and see only the HMO's patients.

Group model is characterized by a group of physicians who contract with the HMO to provide services for a fixed monthly rate per enrollee (capitated rate), but are not HMO employees.

Independent Practice Association (IPA) model is a legal entity sponsored by physicians that contracts with HMOs and are bound by the terms of that contract. The physicians have their own practice and see their own patients as well as care for the HMO's enrollees at the HMO contract rate.

The IPA negotiates with the HMO for payment by a capitated fee or a discounted, fee-for-service rate.

Network model is one in which the HMO contracts directly with IPAs, medical groups and independent physicians forming a provider network. Provider payments are by a capitated fee or a discounted, fee-for-service rate.

Gatekeeper

Gatekeeper is a primary care physician who oversees, authorizes, and coordinates patient medical care that is outside their own practice. Healthcare beyond the gatekeeper must be approved in order to be reimbursed. Gatekeepers are a cost control mechanism as well as means of directing patients to "in-network" providers. True medical or surgical emergencies and routine gynecological care are exempt from gatekeeper referrals.

PPO

PPO, preferred provider organizations, is a large group of medical providers providing medical services on a negotiated or discounted fee-for-service schedule. Enrollees pay a higher coinsurance if they receive services outside the PPO.

EPO

EPO, exclusive provider organizations, use a network of contracted physicians who care for enrollees at a discounted rate. Enrollees are not reimbursed for care received from a provider not part of the EPO.

POS

POS, point of service, plans are a combination of PPO and HMO plan using a contracted network of providers and a primary care physician as gatekeeper to control specialty referrals.

Reimbursements for care provided by out of network physicians are subject to higher deductibles and coinsurance amounts.

Pros and cons of capitation

Capitation is a fee scenario where the provider and managed care organization predict the expenses and revenue of a population group then set a rate for the number of lives covered rather than the services provided. The provider receives a set amount of money each month based on the number of patients in the program, not the number seen for services. The provider purchases reinsurance or stop-loss insurance to cover catastrophic cases. Capitation is seen as a means of cost control, focusing on preventative services to identify early and reduce the expense of catastrophic illness. Criticism of capitation is aimed at physicians who will/do not refer patients for extensive tests or under-treat patients. Physicians may also focus more on fee-for-service patients, which causes patients to question the motivation of the physician to properly treat them.

Regulatory and licensing issues have been raised since physicians are acting as the insurer. Capitation has demonstrated a decrease in the need and cost of specialty services. It has increased the availability of preventative services and early detection of disease while stopping physicians from over-treating patients. It enhances a physician's cash flow.

COB

When someone has more than one health insurance plan, coordination of payments must be done so that no more than 100% of the cost of medical care is reimbursed. Any insurance plan that does not contain COB (Coordination of benefits) provisions must pay for medical care first to avoid overpayment of fees. The following rules apply to COB:

- Employee insurance plans pay first
- A plan that covers the individual as a dependent pays second
- If a dependent covered by multiple plans, the employee with the first birth date is the plan that pays first, only if both plans use the birthday rule and the parents are married
- If the plans do not use the birthday rule and the parents are married, the male parent's plan pays first
- When parents are divorced, the court-appointed primary responsible parent's plan pays first
- When parents are divorced and there is no court determined primary responsible parent, then the plan of the custodial parent pays first followed by the plan of the spouse of the custodial parent followed by the plan of the parents without custody and finally the plan of the spouse of the parent without custody
- Active employee plans pay before in-active (retired) employee plans
- Plans covering an individual as an employee or a dependent pay before a COBRA plan

- If none of the previous rules determine the order of payment, then the plan in place for the longest time pays first

Medical necessity for procedures/treatments

Insurance companies have Medical Directors (state licensed physicians) who oversee claims and determine benefit eligibility for treatment/procedures. The following are procedures followed to document whether or not the facts of the case present a medical necessity.

Foremost, policies must clearly state that medical necessity must be shown for procedures/treatments. Subscribers must have a clear expectation of coverage. If benefits are denied, this is done only following review by the medical director.

Denials should never be based on a monetary incentive. Cases involving high risk procedures (e.g. transplants) or infants in intensive care or oncology wards should have closer review by the medical director, risk manager and possibly corporate counsel. Medical directors should seek guidance from specialists for cases that are outside their area of expertise.

To gain a complete clinical picture, medical directors should speak with the attending physician. Medical directors must carefully document their reviews of medical records, including time and date of the review of each piece of information.

The company should maintain a database of denials in order to assure consistency and a regular review of legal cases will assist in avoiding unwarranted denials.

Viatical settlement

A Case Manager works with many people who are terminally ill or draining their finances in order to cope with an illness. Viatical settlements are a means of obtaining cash out of a person's assets.

Life insurance policies have a cash value at death. To obtain the cash value before death, you can sell the policy at a discount, usually 50% to 85% of the face value depending on your life expectancy, to a company that will collect the face value when you die.

Non-traditional or supplemental policies

Non-traditional or supplemental policies provide comprehensive coverage for a wide range of treatments. These policies include disease-specific policies covering cancer or Alzheimer's, long-term care or nursing home policies, occupational-specific policies (e.g. model insuring their hands/legs), as well as Medigap, dental and vision policies.

Case Manager and a payer's claims department relationship

There are many personnel involved in making claims payments and following the contract language in enforcing benefits. Customer service representatives are the first contact a person has for explanations of eligibility, coverage, and plan specifics. Claims are put into the payer system by a claims processor. Decisions on whether to approve, investigate, or deny claims is made by a claims examiner, usually the next job rung from a claims processor.

Claims supervisors oversee the work flow of both processors and examiners and comprise the first level of management decision making. Final decisions regarding claims are usually the responsibility of the claims manager, although directors and vice presidents will be involved when unique situations arise or litigation might result. The plan administrator handles appeals, plan design and changes to a plan. If the plan is self-funded, one management-level person provides stop-loss advisories.

Case Managers may be involved in discussions between stop-loss carriers and the claims department liaison. The account manager handles service issues, complaints and funding issues.

"Red flag" for payers

A "red flag" is an indication that the case is not routine and will usually benefit from the services of a Case Manager. Different types of insurance require different definitions of red flags. Workers' compensation claims often use lost-time at work guidelines for red flags.

Catastrophic illnesses are red flags for group medical insurance plans, as are premature births or chronic and devastating long-term illnesses. Multiple hospitalizations and multiple physicians are a red flag indicator that extenuating circumstances, beyond the admitting diagnosis, are in existence and may benefit from case management.

The types of services ordered are also a red flag indicator of cases that may benefit from case management. Case Managers work with insurance claims departments to uncover potentially serious cases. Curiosity, instinct and a paper trail are the clues to streamlining medical care and cost containment measures.

Alternate or Extra-contractual Benefit Plans

Insurance plans can have limitations or exclusions that may hinder the most efficient and cost effective medical care. Case Managers may see cost reduction benefits in care that would not be covered under the patient's insurance plan.

Case Managers need to prepare a report clearly stating the benefits and cost reductions in allowing extra-contractual benefits. They need to communicate with the insurer and obtain approval by the payer and knowledge of the approval received by the claims adjuster, prior to the implementation of the care/program. Obtaining extra-contractual benefits is one part of maximizing resources at the patient's disposal.

Knowledge Domains and Subdomains

"Essential functions of a job"

ADA employment provisions are applied only to "qualified individuals," those who have the skill, experience, education and ability to perform essential job functions, with or without reasonable accommodation, as outlined in the job description or collective bargaining agreement. The job functions must be documented before advertising and interviewing applicants, the functions must occupy the majority of the job's time, and they must be required of other people performing the same or similar jobs.

Reasonable accommodations

Reasonable accommodations are modifications to existing facilities making them usable or accessible to an individual with disabilities, e.g. ramp into a doorway or lowering a counter. Accommodating an individual following many injuries or illnesses may not be possible (depression, anger, muscular or cardiovascular endurance) and will require individual analysis and documentation by the Case Manager. Some employers, including religious or private membership organizations, federal government, Native American tribes or employers with fewer than 15 employees, are exempt from the ADA.

Life care plan

A life care plan is a comprehensive overview of the lifetime care of a patient based on clinical and financial information. A full analysis and narrative report of the current and future needs of a patient are included. Acquisition, replacement, repair and upgrading of medical services and items are included at current costs; a medical economist projects and adjusts them for inflation and financial trends. The life care plan is used in the court system as the groundwork for settlements in claims for personal injury or medical liability cases. The current and projected costs and utilization in the following areas must be included in the life care plan: financial status of the patient, medical, psychological, physical and vocational rehabilitation, pharmaceutical and medical supply needs, social support resources, housing needs or architectural modifications, transportation needs, and prosthesis and assistive device needs.

Alternative or complementary care treatments

Case Managers must be aware of all the healthcare options within their community in order to address the unique needs of a large, culturally diverse population. Alternative or complementary care treatments incorporate the concept of mind/body/spirit treatment, holistic medicine and Eastern medicine. Some of these techniques may be administered within and combined with "normal" healthcare (massage during childbirth; prayer circle visiting a patient in a hospital), some may be administered in alternative healthcare facilities (chiropractic care, massage and Reiki), and others are part of a growing alternative healthcare industry (guided imagery, dietary therapy, spiritual healing, herbal remedies, homeopathic treatments, tai chi and yoga).

There are also many treatment facilities for teenagers offering residential and experimental programs.

CARF

CARF is the Commission on Accreditation of Rehabilitation Facilities which sets the criteria for achieving quality care at rehabilitation provider locations. Case Managers should strive to recommend treatment at facilities that are accredited by CARF to assure the quality of care.

NCQA

NCQA is the National Committee on Quality Assurance which oversees the quality of care provided by healthcare organizations and managed care organizations. This designation allows the Case Manager to know that the care group has met predetermined standards.

HEDIS

HEDIS is the Health Plan Employer Data and Information Set which is a collection of standardized performance measures sponsored, supported and maintained by the NCQA, which assist employers and other purchases in the evaluation of health plan operations.

Short-term and long-term disability plan

Disability plans provide income replacement for a prescribed period of time when an individual cannot work due to illness or injury. These are wage replacement plans and lack benefits for medical services. Disability plans are often an optional benefit offered by employers or self-procured by an individual.

Short-term disability (STD) benefits may progress into long-term disability (LTD) benefits or total disability. There are two unique provisions of LTD policies:
- HISOCC (his occupation) refers to all functions required in the person's job. If the person can perform 4 out of 5 job tasks, they still qualify for LTD benefits and collect their full salary for a specified time ranging from 1 to 5 years
- ANYOCC (any occupation) acknowledges a person may not be able to perform all their job tasks, but may be able to perform tasks required in other occupations
- ANYOCC coverage is expensive and provides all or partial salary until a person reaches age 65

Centers for Medicare and Medicaid Services (CMS)

CMS (previously known as the Healthcare Financing Administration-HCFA) is a federal agency that runs the Medicare and Medicaid programs providing benefits to over 75 million Americans. It also covers the State Children's Health Insurance Program (SCHIP).

CMS also has responsibility to regulate laboratory testing on humans (except research) and along with the departments of Labor and Treasury, assists in maintaining health insurance coverage for small companies and individuals and eliminating discrimination based on health status for people purchasing health insurance. CMS combats fraud and abuse in cooperation with federal departments and state and local governments. CMS helps improve the quality of healthcare for people receiving health coverage via its programs through development and enforcement of standards, measuring and improving outcomes of care, and educating healthcare providers and beneficiaries.

Coordination with social programs

Many recipients of Medicaid are underinsured and economically disadvantaged and are coping with life problems that are not related to their illness. This population contains the elderly as well as families who are unemployed or underemployed. The biggest challenge is keeping the patients enrolled in a plan to can provide coordinated services. Finding health providers who will accept Medicaid is one problem, however, basic human needs are often the most pressing problem: obtaining food, housing, clothing and transportation.

Case Managers must be able to identify clinical as well as social needs and work in tandem with social workers when applicable. Arranging meals-on-wheels or homemaker assistance for the elderly, coordinating transportation to/from appointments, and referrals to community services are often handled by Case Managers, even though these services may be out of the normal range of activities done by the Case Manager.

Managed Care Case Manager

Managed care is a financial system developed as a cost containment system in the healthcare industry. Managed care organizations (MCO) have a Case Manager who oversees the care given a patient in order to prevent costs from running over the amount allocated for the disease/treatment.

An MCO Case Manager may need to provide pre-authorization for hospital admittance or for treatment options of clients with developmental disabilities, substance abuse problems or mental health issues. Managed care is an economic system and thus could be at odds with the individualized plan for your client, or the MCO may require their Case Manager be the only Case Manager for your client.

Practice Test

Practice Questions

1. The five components of a nursing case management framework identified by the American Nurses Credentialing Center are:
   a. planning, organizing, coordinating, advocacy, and monitoring
   b. assessment, planning, implementation, evaluation, and interaction
   c. communication, planning, facilitation, advocacy, and monitoring
   d. evaluation, linking, coordination, advocacy, and monitoring

2. The "Pareto Principle," as related to nursing case management, indicates that:
   a. resource allocation must be multidisciplinary to be cost effective
   b. a systematic and dynamically adaptable framework is required
   c. about 80% of all health resources are used by 20% of the population
   d. no professional discipline owns the practice of case management

3. Client assessment in case management is best described as:
   a. completion of a thorough physical exam to identify all health issues
   b. interviews of collateral contacts to understand the client better
   c. a thorough client interview to evaluate identified needs
   d. an in-depth evaluation, including interviews and record reviews

4. Case management systems should be adapted to accommodate all of the following EXCEPT the:
   a. political or cultural views of the case manager
   b. organizational setting in which the services are provided
   c. socioeconomic needs of the population being served
   d. developmental characteristics of the clients being seen

5. A pediatric theorist who focused on the social environment of children is:
   a. B. F. Skinner
   b. Alfred Adler
   c. Erik Erickson
   d. Jean Piaget

6. A financial evaluation is completed for all of the following reasons EXCEPT to:
   a. identify available resources for health care and stability
   b. determine the client's eligibility for case management services
   c. ensure any requisite preapprovals for proposed health care treatments and services.
   d. assist a client and family to apply for additional benefits that may be necessary for heath care needs

7. If a necessary medical treatment or service is denied to a patient, a case manager's options include all of the following EXCEPT:
    a. misconstruing the client's financial status to meet benefit eligibility
    b. requesting a benefit plan exception for circumstances of hardship
    c. seeking community resources to provide coverage as needed
    d. advocating for a longer stay to meet patient needs, pending the availability of other options

8. Implementation of a plan of care involves all the following EXCEPT:
    a. goal setting
    b. negotiation
    c. contracting
    d. delegation

9. The tendency of health care professionals to work in "silos" means:
    a. having a multidisciplinary perspective and appreciation
    b. referring clients to other providers as needed
    c. working independently and without collaboration
    d. accepting and receiving consultation as needed

10. Polypharmacy is best defined as:
    a. having medications dispensed from more than one pharmaceutical source
    b. the pharmaceutical compounding of medicinal blends to provide individually tailored medications and dosages
    c. using a team of pharmacists when addressing patient medication issues
    d. using multiple medications in a single patient

11. Appropriate methods of professional and interdisciplinary communication include all of the following EXCEPT:
    a. chart notes
    b. cafeteria consults
    c. telephone discussions
    d. team meetings

12. The process of identifying key issues, understanding each party's perspective, considering possible solutions and outcomes, determining best options, agreeing on contingencies, and monitoring and evaluating outcomes is known as:
    a. critical thinking and problem-solving
    b. brainstorming and collaboration
    c. program evaluation and implementation
    d. goal setting and assessment

13. The process of establishing patient goals, continuously gathering provider information, measuring progress, and modifying interventions as needed is called:
    a. evaluation
    b. outcomes measurement
    c. clinical assessment
    d. monitoring

14. From a case management perspective, the difference between gross savings and net savings with reference to a service plan is:
    a. any savings realized
    b. the sum of all potential charges less realized charges
    c. the inclusion of case management fees.
    d. the difference between costs and benefits

15. The extent to which patient behavior follows the recommendations of a health care provider is referred to as:
    a. care plan concurrence
    b. patient adherence
    c. treatment synergy
    d. protocol attention

16. Factors that influence a case manager's approach to a case include all of the following EXCEPT:
    a. case manager fees
    b. community resources
    c. payer systems
    d. referral sources

17. The greatest portion of health care costs and resources is directed to:
    a. perinatal and pediatric care issues
    b. geriatric care issues
    c. traumatic accidents and injuries
    d. chronic diseases in all age-groups

18. Disease management programs primarily focus on the:
    a. insurance costs of a particular disease
    b. research on a particular disease
    c. pathophysiological components of a disease
    d. funding options for a particular disease

19. When dealing with the psychosocial aspects of chronic illness, the nurse case manager should do all of the following EXCEPT:
    a. assume the role of therapist for the client and family
    b. listen and learn about the impact of the illness on the client and family
    c. empower clients and families to develop coping strategies
    d. provide referrals to support groups and social services

20. Discovering, respecting, and incorporating the values of clients and families in the health care experience refers to:
    a. sociodemographic tolerance
    b. cultural competence
    c. individuality integration
    d. psychosocial acknowledgment

21. Medical practice standards and care algorithms are often referred to as:
    a. clinical practice guidelines
    b. best practices or clinical protocols
    c. care pathways or care maps
    d. all of the above

22. The health education "Stages of Change Model" was developed by:
    a. Diniz, Schmidt, and Stothers
    b. Malcolm Knowles
    c. James Prochaska
    d. Hildegarde Peplau

23. The 1966 "Partnership for Health Act" defined health as:
    a. a state of complete well-being
    b. an interdisciplinary enterprise
    c. a case management outcome
    d. the promotion of wellness

24. The fundamental starting point for a case manager and patient is:
    a. an understanding of the patient's disease or injury
    b. an appreciation of the patient's sociocultural situation
    c. a holistic understanding of the patient in all life dimensions
    d. diagnostic clarity and a medically effective care plan

25. The term "least restrictive setting" refers to:
    a. the voluntary nature of patient–provider health care delivery
    b. a "start low and go slow" approach to treatment
    c. protocols regarding the use of patient physical restraints
    d. treatment in settings that promote maximal patient autonomy

26. Health information and identified demographics of a single person are referred to as:
    a. individual data
    b. personal data
    c. singular data
    d. prime data

27. Health information and demographics gathered by repeated measurements or by combining a collection of individual data are referred to as:
    a. population data
    b. cumulative data
    c. aggregate data
    d. collective data

28. Quality data have all of the following characteristics EXCEPT they are:
    a. predictable
    b. reliable
    c. unbiased
    d. valid

29. Health care "registries" are defined as:
    a. systems used to admit patients to a health care facility
    b. systems used to collect and follow patient information
    c. case management billing programs
    d. computer-operated waiting lists

30. The difference between computer application programs and system software is best described by which of the following statements?
    a. System software operates a computer's internal systems, while application programs provide the user with a directly applied service
    b. System software provides the user with an applied service, while application programs operate the computer's internal systems
    c. System software is provided to many computers through an organization's computer network, while application programs operate on a single computer
    d. System software operates on a single computer, while application programs are provided to many computers through an organization's computer network

31. Data analysis is defined as:
    a. mathematical calculations, using recognized algorithms and methods
    b. an examination of data to derive useful information
    c. the computerized manipulation of data in an organized fashion
    d. the collection and aggregation of data into a database

32. A histogram is a type of:
    a. pie chart
    b. scattergram
    c. monogram
    d. bar graph

33. Data mining refers to:
    a. data collection derived from underground geological projects
    b. the process of drawing relevant data from a larger data set
    c. the entering of specific data into a specific computer database
    d. data analysis that uses a hidden or background computer program

34. Root-cause analysis refers to:
    a. a search for causal factors producing a given outcome or result
    b. a method of chi-square analysis used to manipulate data
    c. a computer "subroutine" or "root" program used to analyze data
    d. the logistic regression of data against an identified data point

35. Common forms of statistical analyses include all of the following EXCEPT:
    a. hypothesis testing
    b. correlation and regression analysis
    c. kurtosis modeling
    d. confidence interval calculation

36. The theorist who first identified the hierarchy of needs, including (1) physiological needs; (2) safety; (3) love and belonging; (4) self-esteem; and (5) self-actualization, by which to achieve satisfaction and fulfillment was:
    a. Carl Jung
    b. Erik Erickson
    c. Jean Piaget
    d. Abraham Maslow

37. Bower and Falk (1996) defined effective resource management as:
    a. doling out material goods assessed as essential for client health and well-being
    b. coordinating the delivery of targeted goods and services identified by medical providers as necessary for client recovery from illness or injury
    c. identifying, confirming, coordinating, and negotiating resources to meet client needs
    d. determining the most efficient and cost-effective method of service and resource delivery to meet a client's health and recovery needs

38. Three nationwide referral resources for senior services include which of the following?
    a. Eldercare Locator, Snap for Seniors, and the 211 telephone information and referral
    b. Just for Seniors, Senior Connections, and the Golden Lions
    c. Grey Panthers, American Association of Retired Persons, and Senior Living
    d. Senior Connections, Retired Referrals, and Elder Advantage

39. All of the following are social service agencies that can assist case managers in obtaining community resources for their patients EXCEPT:
    a. Centers for Medicaid eligibility
    b. Centers for Independent Living
    c. Department of Social Services
    d. Agency on Aging.

40. Free or low-cost vaccinations, health screenings, health education classes, tracking and reporting of communicable diseases and collection of local health statistics for prevention and regulatory programs are all functions typically carried out by:
    a. acute care hospitals
    b. public health services
    c. urgent care clinics
    d. health insurers

41. The 1975 federal Education for All Handicapped Children Act requires all of the following EXCEPT:
    a. free public education with equal opportunity for handicapped children
    b. the development of proper evaluation and classification procedures
    c. individualized education programs based on evaluation
    d. private in-home education based on disability severity

42. Vocational services are primarily intended to assist individuals who have sustained a catastrophic illness or injury with:
   a. socialization skills to develop interpersonal relationships
   b. in-home activities of daily living for personal independence
   c. employment that accommodates physical and mental challenges
   d. the achievement of self-actualized goals and aspirations

43. The five basic "levels of care" in the health care system include which of the following?
   a. acute, subacute, custodial, assisted living, and outpatient
   b. acute, subacute, custodial, home, and outpatient
   c. acute, subacute, custodial, private nursing, and outpatient
   d. acute, subacute, hospice, custodial, and outpatient

44. The three broadest definitions of health care supplies and equipment are:
   a. ambulation aids, pill dispensers, and wound care products
   b. personal care aids, dressings, and pharmaceuticals
   c. durable medical equipment, disposables, and pharmaceuticals
   d. disposables, durable equipment, and personal care products

45. When ordering durable medical equipment, case managers should also ensure all of the following EXCEPT that the:
   a. equipment arrives in working order
   b. patient and caregiver know how to use it properly
   c. training for safety and maintenance is completed
   d. warranties and manufacturers' data are included

46. The most significant difference between "utilization review" and "utilization management" is:
   a. utilization review is conducted solely to determine insurance contract compliance, while utilization management is conducted for purposes of cost containment
   b. utilization review is carried out by clinicians for quality control, while utilization management is carried out by facility administrators
   c. utilization review is retrospective, while utilization management is oriented toward the present and future
   d. utilization review is a clerical task, while utilization management is an administrative task

47. A patient is facing an upcoming surgical procedure, but his coverage for the procedure is not clear. Week's after filing a written request, the insurer has still has not provided clarification. The procedure is now becoming unduly delayed. The best case management response would be to:
   a. write further letters to various administrators at the company
   b. file a grievance with the appropriate oversight agency
   c. perform the procedure and request coverage later
   d. advise the client to hire an attorney to press the matter

48. An individual has Medicaid coverage, and the case manager is having difficulty finding a provider who is willing to provide needed health care for Medicaid-only payment rates. The case manager's best option is to:
   a. contact the local Medicaid field office for consultation
   b. negotiate for the patient to pay additional out-of-pocket costs
   c. call the local physician's licensing board to complain
   d. tell the patient to seek alternate insurance options

49. Three kinds of utilization review include:
   a. clerical, clinical, and research review
   b. coverage, cost, and quality review
   c. preauthorization, concurrent, and retrospective review
   d. resource, utilization, and quality-control–based review

50. A managed care provider has denied payment for a specific procedure. An appeal may then subsequently be submitted, providing additional documentation. Denial of services is always provided by a:
   a. nurse
   b. clerk
   c. business manager
   d. physician

51. TRICARE refers to a:
   a. cardiac catheterization procedure
   b. government insurance plan
   c. multilayer nursing care system
   d. subacute care facility

52. The acronyms HMO, PPO, and POS all refer to:
   a. private health insurance plans
   b. methods of cost-benefit analysis
   c. clinical quality outcome indicators
   d. evidence-based medical measures

53. The term "subrogation" refers to:
   a. payment by a secondary insurer after primary insurance benefits have been exhausted
   b. benefit negotiations between patients, physicians, and insurers
   c. medical expense reimbursement of an insurer or self-insured employer out of a third-party settlement
   d. subcontracting medical care services to a third-party provider

54. The Prospective Pay System bases medical services reimbursement on:
   a. the client's ability to pay for the services rendered
   b. usual and customary fees as billed by other practitioners
   c. average fees as billed in a given geographic area
   d. predetermined rates for diagnostic-related groups

55. The best definition of "benchmarking" is the:
    a. calibration of medical machinery to ensure accurate and consistent performance
    b. comparison of products, services, and practices among different providers or leaders in a given specialty
    c. analysis of data to produce a baseline performance index for purposes of outcomes comparisons
    d. compilation of recent performance data into a standardized format for later analysis

56. The Quality Improvement Organization program is operated under the auspices of the:
    a. Centers for Medicare and Medicaid Services
    b. Joint Commission
    c. National Quality Forum
    d. National Committee for Quality Assurance

57. An "ombudsman" is best described as:
    a. an accreditation analyst who evaluates health care organizations, programs, and policies
    b. an independent official who arbitrates health care disputes and levies sanctions and fines where required
    c. a neutral source of assistance to address the health care service concerns of local citizens
    d. an insurance investigator who resolves health care coverage and benefit issues

58. Best practice profiling in health care can best be described as the:
    a. evaluation of various services within a single specialty to determine the most effective system of health care delivery
    b. intensive evaluation of a health care service, function, or organization for quality outcomes indicators
    c. comparison of relevant benchmark data to determine services, processes, or functions that produce superior outcomes
    d. identification of errors and obstacles that impede quality health care services, functions, and programs

59. The five fundamental steps of evidence-based practice include all of the following EXCEPT:
    a. evaluating and then applying the evidence located
    b. problem identification and literature/resource review
    c. re-examination of the outcomes and revising as needed
    d. varying the techniques used for optimum results

60. The most likely cause for "variance" in a clinical pathway (i.e., deviation from an expected pattern on a clinical pathway) is:
    a. patient noncompliance
    b. practitioner variation
    c. health care system deviation
    d. all of the above

61. Continuous quality improvement (CQI) requires all of the following to achieve a stated goal or aim EXCEPT:
    a. a fully defined goal and enough time to achieve it
    b. a CQI "champion" or leader to mobilize others
    c. good working relationships and "buy-in" from team members and administration
    d. approval of the goal from accreditation or credentialing programs

62. As related to continuous quality improvement, the acronym "PDSA" stands for:
    a. prepare, direct, summarize, and anticipate
    b. plan, do, study, and act
    c. postulate, disseminate, schedule, and articulate
    d. propose, discuss, situate, and align

63. A. The acronyms DMAIC and DMADV refer to quality-improvement sub-methodologies used within which of the following models?
    a. Shewhart cycle
    b. Continuous quality improvement
    c. Six sigma model
    d. Deming cycle

64. In the field of quality improvement, the term "core measures" refers to:
    a. National Quality Forum standards for quality control in health care
    b. specific Centers for Medicare and Medicaid Services–required quality-control measures
    c. Joint Commission criteria for quality improvement
    d. health provider–selected quality-improvement measures

65. The purpose of the National Quality Forum is to:
    a. ensure that health care facilities remain clean
    b. set standards for business tax compliance
    c. monitor infection control policies
    d. provide standardized health care quality measures

66. The main difference between "quality management" and "risk management" is:
    a. problem prevention versus problem analysis and liability control
    b. clinical practice versus business management standards
    c. practicum-based versus policy-based models of care
    d. care provider versus administration-oriented standards

67. Empathy with the patient, understanding resistance, identifying patient readiness to change, and clear and honest communication are all safeguards to ensure ethical case manager behavior during the process of:
    a. negotiation
    b. treatment
    c. interviewing
    d. motivating

68. The ethical principal of autonomy is best defined as:
    a. readiness for change
    b. do no harm
    c. self-determination
    d. individual responsibility

69. The difference between confidentiality and privacy is best described as:
    a. information protection versus personal revelation
    b. personal seclusion versus controlled information release
    c. legal access versus limited exposure
    d. authorized access versus the right to self-disclose

70. Aside from the issue of insurance portability, the primary purpose of the Health Insurance Portability and Accountability Act of 1996 was to:
    a. ensure peer review of health care practices
    b. protect private health information
    c. address health care billing practices
    d. set standards for quality review

71. The Health Insurance Portability and Accountability Act of 1966 grants individuals the right to all of the following EXCEPT:
    a. copies of health records and notices about how health information will be used and shared
    b. corrections added to the health information, and reports about why health information was shared in certain situations
    c. the option to give or refuse permission for information sharing, such as for marketing or certain other purposes
    d. deletion or removal of negative personal health information from a treating provider's records

72. The best definition for when a "living will" becomes effective is when:
    a. decisional capacity is lost
    b. a person is terminally ill or permanently unconscious
    c. a physician feels that the document should be "invoked"
    d. further treatment appears to be futile

73. Medical "assault" (e.g., the threat or attempt to render medical care over a patient's objections), medical "battery" (e.g., physical contact of a person without consent), and "false imprisonment" (e.g., inappropriate use of restraints) are all best defined as:
    a. civil infractions of the law
    b. criminal conduct
    c. intentional torts
    d. penal code violations

74. Medical "invasion of privacy" (e.g., taking digital images of a patient without consent, breaking confidentiality) and "defamation of character" (e.g., verbally delivered false or malicious statements that injure a person's reputation, such as pejorative statements about a patient in an elevator; falsehoods or malicious and damaging communications in writing, print, signs, or pictures, such as pejorative chart notes, that damage a person's reputation) are both examples of:
    a. statutory violations
    b. criminal conduct
    c. civil code infractions
    d. quasi-intentional torts

75. Medical "malpractice" (i.e., failure to respond as a "reasonable and prudent professional," resulting in harm) and "negligence" (i.e., failing to act as any "reasonable and prudent" person in a given circumstance independent of any professional context, as the failure does not address training or special skills) are both examples of:
    a. unintentional torts
    b. intentional negligence
    c. unintentional misconduct
    d. quasi-malpractice

76. Medical "abandonment" is best defined as:
    A. failure to render necessary medical treatment due to deliberate neglect
    B. an unintentional oversight of requisite care from which harm resulted
    C. the willful failure to be responsible for a person for whom one has a care giving duty
    d. the unavoidable and unintentional absence of a caregiver resulting in harm.

77. Stress can motivate learning. The most rapid learning occurs at which of the following stress levels?
    a. Low stress
    b. Low-to-moderate stress
    c. Moderate-to-high stress
    d. High stress

78. Reinforcement is the process of encouraging correct behavior and discouraging incorrect behavior. When using reinforcement, an educator should:
    a. emphasize positive reinforcement strategies
    b. focus on extinguishing negative behaviors
    c. use both positive and negative reinforcement strategies
    d. avoid any emphasis on either positive or negative behaviors

79. In educational experiences, information retention is most directly affected by the:
    a. degree to which the information presented is entertaining
    b. simplicity and clarity of the language used in the presentation
    c. level to which the information presented is personally relevant
    d. amount of practice incorporated into the learning experience

80. Malcolm Knowles' theory of "andragogy" includes which of the following three key characteristics of the adult learner?
   a. Self-direction, learning readiness, and a problem-centered orientation to learning
   b. Autonomy, self-direction, and a life-experience orientation to learning
   c. Practicality, goal-orientation, and respect
   d. Life-experience, practicality, and self-direction

81. Researchers have categorized which of the following three general information learning styles?
   a. Auditory, visual, and kinesthetic
   b. Perceptual modality, information processing, and personality patterns
   c. Direct, ancillary and incidental, and multimodal based
   d. Integrative, associative, and perceptive

82. Perceptions of health, illness, disease, healing, and wellness are most influenced by:
   a. family and religion
   b. gender and income
   c. culture and language
   d. age and education

83. The capacity to understand and use health care information is most strongly influenced by:
   a. gender
   b. marital status
   c. ethnicity
   d. literacy

84. For non-English-speaking patients, a "medical interpreter" differs from a "medical translator" in which of the following ways?
   a. An interpreter works with spoken language, and a translator deals with written language
   b. A translator deals with spoken language, and an interpreter deals with written language
   c. A medical interpreter addresses specific treatments and procedures, and a medical translator deals with nonmedical issues
   d. A medical translator addresses specific treatments and procedures, and a medical interpreter deals with nonmedical issues

85. The American Nurses Association has identified all but one of the following as the "Six Standards of Practice"?
   a. Interview, identify, plan, intervene, monitor, and evaluate
   b. Listen, diagnose, treat, evaluate, report, and revise
   c. Examine, consult, diagnose, plan, implement, and evaluate
   d. Assess, diagnose, identify outcomes, plan, implement, and evaluate

86. Case management standards are set by the various disciplines involved (social workers and nurses) as well as by the Case Management Society of America. The standards are further supported by:
    a. application criteria
    b. measurement guidelines
    c. practice outlines
    d. intervention definitions

87. The terms "licensure" and "certification" are sometimes used interchangeably, but they actually differ in which of the following ways?
    a. Licensure is evidence of merely attending a program of training, while certification refers to a process of examination and performance
    b. Certification is evidence of merely attending a program of training, while licensure refers to a process of examination and performance
    c. Licensure is a legal form of professional validation, while certification refers to competence in a specialized area of a profession
    d. Certification is a legal form of professional validation, while licensure refers to competence in a specialized area of a profession

88. Milliman care guidelines and InterQual differ in purpose primarily in which of the following ways?
    a. Milliman addresses utilization review, while InterQual addresses quality-control issues
    b. Milliman addresses treatment guidelines, while InterQual addresses the continuum of care
    c. Milliman offers guidelines, while InterQual mandates care criteria
    d. Milliman is used by clinicians, while InterQual is used by insurers

89. Health screening tools are categorized in which of the following three ways?
    a. Self-administered, interview-based, and integrated
    b. Descriptive, quantitative, and qualitative
    c. Descriptive, evaluative, and predictive
    d. Scaled, aggregate, and discrete

90. The most common screening tool in managed care and among health care providers is the:
    a. functional living index
    b. mini-mental status examination
    c. Hopkins symptom checklist 25
    d. short-form 36 health survey

91. Statements that are systematically developed to aid health providers and patients to determine appropriate health care options in defined clinical circumstances are known as:
    a. clinical practice guidelines
    b. standards of practice
    c. care delivery standards
    d. care algorithms

92. A flowchart format of health care decisions that target a specific health condition, along with treatment processes, care sequences, and usually including an expected medical course, is referred to as a:
    a. medical flowchart
    b. diagnostic tree
    c. clinical pathway
    d. practice guideline

93. Algorithms and protocols are similar and dissimilar in which of the following ways?
    a. Algorithms are applied in treatment situations, but protocols are applied in care coordination decisions
    b. They are both treatment oriented, but protocols are supported by scientific data
    c. There is no difference between algorithms and care protocols
    d. They both use stepwise sequencing, but algorithms are supported by research-based data

94. Clinical "decision trees" are most frequently used when:
    a. a situation does not clearly present a best course of action
    b. a clinician is relatively inexperienced
    c. a specialist is not available in an urgent situation
    d. numerous comorbidities are present

95. Consumer Assessment of Healthcare Provider and Systems consumer satisfaction surveys are administered under the auspices of the:
    a. Joint Commission
    b. Centers for Medicare and Medicaid Services
    c. National Quality Forum
    d. Agency for Health Care Research and Quality

96. The Case Management Society of America was founded in:
    a. 1985
    b. 1990
    c. 1993
    d. 1995

97. Case management preceptorship and mentoring differ in which of the following ways?
    a. Preceptorship is formal and supervisory, while mentoring is informal and is less instructional
    b. Preceptors work with experienced staff, while mentors work exclusively with those new to the field
    c. Preceptors are members of academia, while mentors are actively working case managers
    d. Preceptors are working case managers, while mentors are members of academia

98. When an organization offers training, in-services, orientation to new laws, and other opportunities for employees or contract providers to obtain new skills and knowledge, it is formally referred to as:
    a. continuing education
    b. credentialing
    c. tuition reimbursement
    d. staff development

99. Three essential tools for employee/contractee evaluation are:
    a. mentor, preceptor, and supervisor/contractor discussions
    b. agency satisfaction surveys, informal discussions, and staff meetings
    c. performance appraisals, peer review, and self-evaluation
    d. colleague consults, in-service meetings, and continuing education

100. The responsibility for a licensed or certified professional to remain current in knowledge, skills, and other professional competencies rests primarily on the:
    a. employer, as a matter of accreditation
    b. licensing/credentialing body that endorsed the individual
    c. professional who holds a license, certification, or credential
    d. state oversight board that ensures consumer protection

Answers and Explanations

1. B: Assessment, planning, implementation, evaluation, and interaction. Nursing case management is a process of meeting an individual's health care needs through collaboration and coordination. It requires assessment to determine client needs, planning to identify and engage resources, timely implementation to reduce service fragmentation, evaluation to ensure quality care and effective clinical outcomes, and interaction in an ongoing fashion to realize all client goals and outcomes.

2. C: About 80% of all health resources are used by 20% of the population. The "Pareto Principle" (also known as the "80–20 rule," the law of the "vital few," and the principle of "factor sparsity") states that, for many real world events, roughly 80% of the effects come from 20% of the causes. Applied to case management, it means that approximately 20% of all patients consume 80% of all medical resources. This resource-intense population must be identified and carefully "case managed" so that their health care is of high quality, efficiently delivered (i.e., meeting expected outcomes), and cost-effective.

3. D: An in-depth evaluation, including interviews and record reviews. Clients identified for case management assessment are at-risk for or in need of intensive services either because of complex health problems or high-resource use. Thus, assessment for purposes of case management involves an in-depth evaluation of a client and his or her complete situation. It incorporates interviews with the client and other relevant sources, along with an intensive review of all pertinent records from health care institutions, involved professionals, employers, caregivers, school and military sources, and health care providers, among others. The goal is to obtain insights into a client's physical, psychosocial, cultural, developmental, economic, lifestyle, and spiritual circumstances sufficient to uncover all significant health care issues.

4. A: Political or cultural views of the case manager. The focus of case management is on optimum client care, regardless of the political, cultural, or other personal views of any given case manager. While broad guidelines for case management are provided by credentialing bodies, the specific features of the case management system used should be tailored to meet the age, function, developmental capabilities, mental illnesses, economics, cultural characteristics, and capacities of the clients who are served and the service delivery organization that is involved.

5. C: Erik Erickson. Erik Erickson's theories incorporated insights into the social environment of children, illuminating issues, such as peer pressure, that may influence their willingness to adhere to prescribed treatment regimens and medication usage. B. F. Skinner emphasized behavioral issues that were treated with rewards, bargaining, and other behavioral modification techniques. Jean Piaget developed cognitive theories of pediatric interaction, clarifying, for example, the need of children for comfort and parental support more than reasoning, explaining, and rationally addressing the need for any given procedure or intervention. Alfred Adler was not a pediatric theorist.

6. B: Determine the client's eligibility for case management services. Clients are referred for case management services based on need, risk, and resource usage, not on their ability to pay for the services. While the extent of services offered may correlate with an ability to pay for those services, financial status is not a prerequisite to case management. A failure to evaluate a client's financial status properly can lead to overlooked resources, services, and even available treatments. Further, failure to complete an evaluation of insurance benefits and coverage may lead to denials of referrals, treatments, and services, and even to costs unnecessarily billed to patients because of a failure to identify, preauthorize, or bill properly for needed treatments and services.

7. A: Misconstruing the client's financial status to meet benefit eligibility. It would be unethical for a case manager to misrepresent (or to coach a client to misrepresent) the client's financial status regardless of cause or need. Such misrepresentation constitutes fraud and can lead to civil and even criminal liability. All other options noted above, however, are within the case manager's purview. Indeed, they are obligations of quality practice and proper client advocacy, as they represent the full development of a patient-centered plan that seeks evidence-based interdisciplinary facilitated outcomes.

8. D: Delegation. A plan that is developed and approved by all involved parties (including the treating physician, the patient and family, and the payer) is not delegated but is implemented by the nurse case manager. While various aspects of treatment and service provision may be delegated to the various disciplines involved, the case manager must not abdicate his or her responsibility to continue the implementation and management of the treatment and service plan. To this end, the case manager uses necessary skills and education in critical thinking, knowledge, evaluation, negotiating, contracting, and decision-making. Goals must be patient-specific and relevant. Negotiation involves building relationships, trust, and flexibility. Contracting is required to engage organizations and vendors to provide the necessary treatments and services.

9. C: Working independently and without collaboration. Professional training has the effect of focusing practitioners primarily on their specialized knowledge base. Thus, there is a natural tendency to practice independently and without collaboration. Consequently, a primary goal of nursing case management is to bring diverse specialties together to address common patient treatment goals and to share unique expertise to meet the identified goals of care. This process of collaboration is primarily carried out by consultation and referral.

10. D: Using multiple medications in a single patient. The situation tends to result from the involvement of multiple physician providers who have little or no interactions with each other and who, thus, prescribe medications without full regard for the other medications the patient is already taking. Polypharmacy situations readily arise in situations of complex chronic conditions and increase the risk of problematic drug interactions, sensitivity, and unanticipated overdose. Issues of unnecessary cost also arise. Competent case managers are uniquely positioned to reduce untoward polypharmacy.

11. B: Cafeteria consults. The phrase "cafeteria consults" suggests communications about privileged patient information in a public setting. Principles of confidentiality require professionals to take reasonable steps to prevent the untoward dissemination of patient information to uninvolved or otherwise inappropriate parties. Other appropriate venues of information sharing include properly directed e-mails and faxes, written narratives,

teleconferences, face-to-face discussions, and multidisciplinary rounds. Accurate information sharing, summarization without distortion, and ethnically and culturally sensitive communication that is tailored to the hearer's educational level is very important.

12. A: Critical thinking and problem-solving. Critical thinking and problem-solving use the processes identified in the question. Successful critical thinking and problem-solving require creativity, flexibility, quality assessment, communication skills, and organizational proficiency. Applying critical thinking and problem-solving skills enables nurse case managers to anticipate and recognize problems before they become overwhelming, develop workable solutions, and maintain high-quality continuity of care.

13. D: Monitoring. Nurse case management involves the monitoring of established plans, their goals, patients' progress, intervention outcomes, and cost and service delivery. When goals are not met, the treatment or intervention plans must be modified. Involved providers must be kept informed about their collaborative role in the treatment process so that they can optimize their services and maximize the benefits to their patients. The monitoring process is integral to the continuous quality improvement required of health care entities for purposes of accreditation, and it formalizes the role of the nurse case manager.

14. C: The inclusion of case management fees. Gross savings can be calculated by subtracting actual charges from the known potential charges realized without case management benefits (i.e., usual costs minus avoided charges, discounts, and negotiated charges). Net savings is defined as gross savings less the fees from case management. Gross savings and net savings are the primary parts of an overall "cost-benefit" analysis.

15. B: Patient adherence. To maximize care plan adherence, health care providers and patients should develop a consensus on what guidelines the patient can and will follow, given issues of lifestyle, treatment burdens, culture, environment, costs, cognitive capacity, and support systems. An important activity of case mangers is to identify issues of noncompliance and any associated barriers to be able to develop alternate care plans, minimizing the barriers and maximizing care plan adherence. This typically involves careful observation, interviewing, motivation mapping, options exploration, teaching, and re-committing the patient to the plan of care.

16. A: Case manager fees. While sliding-scale service fees may be necessary, this fee structure should not influence the case manager's approach to a case. However, available community resources and client eligibility, the benefits available (or limited) through a payer, and the referral source and rationale all can influence a case manager's management of a case. The need to advocate for a client in need of specific service's and/or resources may arise. The case manager remains responsible for quality care and outcomes once a referral has been accepted or a client has been admitted to a facility where case managers provide services.

17. D: Chronic diseases in all age-groups. Chronic conditions consume over 60% of all medical care costs in the United States, and more than 90 million Americans suffer from one or more chronic conditions. Chronic conditions are defined as those conditions that are prolonged in nature and that fail to resolve independently. Because of the disproportionate consumption of resources and high costs, chronic conditions are often in need of case management to reduce their burden on the overall health care system.

18. C: Pathophysiological components of a disease. A thorough understanding of a given disease process better enables the management of the disease and its impact on the patient. To this end, case managers often specialize in certain high-risk diseases. By doing so, they may develop unique insights into the disease, as well as build efficient relationships with necessary providers and organizations that offer optimum treatments and resources. Areas of specialization include organ transplant recipients, AIDS patients, and patients with respiratory conditions, such as asthma and chronic obstructive pulmonary disease.

19. A: Assume the role of therapist for the client and family. While the nurse case manager should be sensitive to the needs of the patient and family, listen and provide support, and understand the impact of the illness or injury on family dynamics, he or she should not attempt to assume a strictly therapeutic role. Instead, referrals should be made to support groups and social services (e.g., counseling, as needed) for any in-depth psychological services. However, staying well informed, monitoring progress, and relaying essential psychosocial information to relevant members of the health care team is a crucial role of the nurse case manager.

20. B: Cultural competence. The term includes the collective influences from religion, ethnicity, age, gender, geography, language, and socioeconomic status. Cultural competence does not ignore the fact that there are always individual differences and idiosyncrasies from one person to another but refers to an underlying awareness and context that can inform and facilitate the process of understanding and working with each individual. Principles of "diversity" acknowledge that "religion" and "spirituality" are not always the same thing (i.e., one implies membership, while the other refers to personal practice and belief) and that variations exist in behavioral norms, rules, beliefs, values, taboos, and habits among people everywhere. Integration of a cultural assessment into the care plan can aid in issues of communication, treatment compliance, and in the identification and resolution of treatment obstacles.

21. D: All of the above. In nursing case management, the term "clinical practice guidelines" is often used, but the other terms listed in the question also appear frequently in nursing and other medical literature. Clinical guidelines attempt to integrate key treatment decisions with optimum outcomes as derived from research-based evidence of the risks, benefits, and costs associated with various clinical options in a given medical scenario. The research used to develop such guidelines must be "evidence-based" and "practice-based" to ensure that effective outcomes and goals are achieved. Existing clinical guidelines must be frequently reviewed and updated (at least annually) to incorporate ongoing learning and new research findings.

22. C: James Prochaska. James Prochaska produced the health education plan, known as "Stages of Change Model," in 1979 and refined it later with Carlo DiClemente. The model summarizes the six stages that people tend to pass through when attempting to introduce changes in their health-related habits. Stage 1 is called the "pre-contemplation" stage: patients are oblivious to or not seriously considering the need for change. Stage 2 is the "contemplation" stage: people are thinking seriously about making a change. Stage 3 is the "preparation" stage: people make formal plans for an impending change. Stage 4 refers to the "action" stage: the plans are now applied. Stage 5 is the "maintenance" stage: people work past lapses to retain the change. Stage 6 is the "termination" stage: relapse tendencies are resolved, and the change is fully incorporated.

23. A: A state of complete well-being. A state of complete well-being includes physical, mental, and social health. The intent of the Partnership for Health Act was to move away from prior definitions of health that focused on an absence of illness or injury. Thus, the goal was revised from providing treatment resources and access in response to illness and injury to the preemptive promotion of wellness to circumvent and prevent illness and injury. This goal remains a work in progress, as health care delivery systems in the United States continue to be oriented toward responding to situations of disease and injury as opposed to preventing them and promoting greater overall health in society.

24. C: A holistic understanding of the patient in all life dimensions. A segmented understanding of a patient's diagnosis, disease, injury treatment protocols, or sociocultural context can never replace a holistic and integrated understanding of a patient in all of his or her personal life domains. For example, every medical insight and treatment advantage may fail if confounding sociocultural factors exist. A holistic view imbues all care plan interventions with greater efficacy and value. From activity logs, to changes in health patterns, to reports of key indices of risk and outcomes, all have greater meaning and import when placed in a holistic patient context.

25. D: Treatment in settings that promote maximal patient autonomy. Historically, patient treatment was provided in settings that optimized a health care provider's convenience and control. Over the years, it was discovered that patients could become overly dependent and even "institutionalized" by such approaches, leaving them unable to function independently or to return to normal life patterns. To counteract this historical mindset, regulations and policies were promulgated that fostered maximal patient autonomy and independence, ultimately benefiting patients, providers, and the institutional care settings.

26. A: Individual data. Health and demographic data pertaining to a single individual consist of information necessary to understand and respond to a patient's health care situation. These data are needed to shape an effective plan of care. Inaccurate, unavailable, or lost information can lead to expensive testing redundancy and associated risks, inaccurate diagnoses, untoward reactions to treatments and interventions, and other adverse outcomes. Consequently, the collection, maintenance, and availability of this information are important.

27. C: Aggregate data. Aggregate data are necessary to identify and understand health care trends, unique issues, and probabilities as related to health changes over time or changes related to targeted groups and populations. Aggregate data can also be used to track the overall effectiveness of various treatment approaches and other health care interventions. Consequently, aggregate data can be extremely important to nurse case managers as they work with their clients and referral sources.

28. A: Predictable. Data need not be predictable (i.e., providing results or findings that are expected). However, quality data must be reliable (i.e., with results that are consistently repeatable in subsequent measurements), unbiased (i.e., free of systematic errors that compromise the information), and valid (i.e., actually measuring what they purport to measure).

29. B: Systems used to collect and follow patient information. They usually include the capacity to aggregate information by patient group, disease, and diagnosis. Examples

include certain electronic medical records, certain electronic health records systems, and some electronic case management systems; however, not all of these systems include registry capacities. Sophisticated registries can only sort patients by specific health status measures (e.g., blood pressure, blood tests), but they also produce reminders for age- and health-specific tests, track treatment compliance, and produce lists of patients by care needs.

30. A: System software operates a computer's internal systems, while application programs provide the user with a directly applied service. Systems software is managed by information technology personnel, such as computer programmers, while computer application programs are used by the individual computer users (case managers). Examples of systems software include file management tools and the computer's operating system (e.g., Windows). Examples of computer application programs include data management programs, such as Access and Excel, along with word processing programs or e-mail programs.

31. B: An examination of data to derive useful information. While data analysis often uses mathematical calculations and frequently involves the use of a computer, these are not adequate definitions of data analysis. Indeed, "qualitative" data are frequently analyzed by descriptive means, and may not include quantitative (mathematical) analysis at all. Finally, while the collection and aggregation of data are relevant to data analysis, they precede the process of analysis and are not typically part of the analysis function.

32. D: Bar graph. A histogram is a kind of bar graph. It uses rectangular-shaped bars to create a graph of a frequency distribution in which rectangles are used to represent a given variable's number of classes and the frequencies of each. The base of the rectangle rests on a horizontal axis and is proportional to the number of classes representing the given variable, and the height (on the vertical axis) corresponds to the frequency reported for each class. The overall relationship of the bar heights to each other denotes the "shape" of the data, with a mounded, center-weighted shape suggesting a more "normal" or "bell-shaped curve." The far left and right areas of such a bell-shaped graph are referred to as "tails," and any tendency of the overall shape to accumulate more toward the overall left or right indicates data that are "skewed" in one direction or another.

33. B: The process of drawing relevant data from a larger data set. Extremely large data sets can address a broad array of variables. Not all variables in a data set are relevant to a specific area of inquiry. Consequently, the data set is "mined" for data that addresses a specific area of interest or concern. When the necessary data have been extracted from the larger data set, they can then be analyzed to derive any possible inferences and conclusions relevant to the questions or concerns examined by the investigator.

34. A: A search for causal factors producing a given outcome or result. This process is frequently used to investigate any deviations from expected outcomes or variations in systems or personnel performance. It is an integral part of any continuous quality improvement program and is essential in health care, where deviations from standard performance patterns or outcomes can signal issues with serious repercussions for patients and providers.

35. C: Kurtosis modeling. Kurtosis modeling is not a form of statistical analysis but is instead a method of describing the shape of graphed data. A kurtosis distribution is referred to as "high" when its graph has a sharp peak and long, fat tails. A kurtosis distribution is referred to as "low" when it has a rounded peak and tails that are short and thin. Hypothesis tests are used to validate or refute a specific postulation. Correlation and regression analyses are used to determine that a given variable can predict or induce changes in another variable. Confidence intervals are used to indicate the probability that a given finding is not the result of an analytical error.

36. D: Abraham Maslow. In his 1943 paper, "A Theory of Human Motivation," Maslow first proposed his theory of hierarchical needs, which was more fully developed in his book, "Motivation and Personality," published in 1954. Understanding the hierarchical nature of human needs can help case managers more effectively focus the services and resources they bring to bear on a given case. Learning about the needs of a patient and determining how best to overcome any barriers and meet these needs is fundamental to effective resource management.

37. C: Identifying, confirming, coordinating, and negotiating resources to meet client needs. Effective resource management requires that the case manager assesses a client's situation and needs, using a multidisciplinary goal-oriented approach. Adequate understanding of the client's situation and his or her needs requires careful listening and observation. Effective case managers also require a repertoire of reliable providers to ensure continuity of care and high-quality outcomes.

38. A: Elder Care Locator, Snap for Seniors, and the 211 telephone information and referral. The number 211 is a 24-hour telephone information and referral source serving communities nationwide through a United Way collaboration. Eldercare Locator (www.eldercare.gov) is a national network of senior care resources. Snap for Seniors (www.snapforseniors.com) is a searchable database of senior services and providers. Another well-known resource for assisting seniors is the "Case Management Resource Guide," which is available as a printed book or online (see: www.cmrg.com). Other referral resources above are either nonexistent agencies, local organizations, or national organizations grouped with one or more other entities that did not meet the full definition provided.

39. A: Centers for Medicaid eligibility. Centers for Medicaid eligibility authorize state-funded medical care coverage. They do not represent local community resources for patients. Centers for Independent Living provide training and transitional support for individuals seeking to regain independent living skills. Local Departments of Social Services can assist with patient assessments, resource identification, and links to services. Area Agency on Aging offices are another setting for resource referrals, along with caregiver and support group referrals, all of which address senior issues.

40. B: Public health services. These state- and locally funded programs operate free or sliding-scale payment clinics where primary care and public health issues are addressed. Well-baby screenings and immunizations, testing for genetic diseases, screening of food, water, and medications to ensure public safety are all functions carried out by public health services and clinics. Other functions include adult inoculations (i.e., flu, pneumonia), health education regarding substance abuse, weight-loss, domestic abuse, and communicable

disease reporting and tracking (e.g., tuberculosis, sexually transmitted diseases, HIV, meningitis). These centers are invaluable resources for case managers.

41. D: Private in-home education based on disability severity. Public education is provided in community settings, not in private in-home settings. However, an individualized education program may recommend that educational endeavors be augmented by student participation in early intervention programs, such as occupational, physical, and speech therapies. Special medical needs may also be accommodated in certain specialized educational settings, such as nursing support and on-site medications management.

42. C: Employment that accommodates physical and mental challenges. The primary goal of vocational services (e.g., education, rehabilitation, medical services) is to assist an individual to return to employment in a work setting that optimizes his or her maximum capacities. This requires ongoing multidisciplinary assessments (e.g., behavioral, functional, aptitude, achievement) to identify individual capacity and "transferable skills" (i.e., when a return to prior work is not possible), as well as professional intervention and work setting trials until optimum potential is achieved.

43. A: Acute, subacute, custodial, assisted living, and outpatient. Acute care settings provide highly skilled hospitalization and acute rehabilitation. Subacute settings address health care delivery beyond what can be met by patients and families in the home but are less intensive than acute settings. Some rehabilitative services, hospice care, skilled nursing home care, and private-duty in-home nursing may meet subacute care standards. Custodial care involves the management of stable but chronic conditions and disabilities for which care cannot be provided in the home. Assisted living allows individuals to maintain personal independence, with support to meet needs that are limited by mobility and stable health problems. Outpatient care is provided in facilities that augment care to those living in residential settings.

44. C: Durable medical equipment, disposables, and pharmaceuticals. Durable medical equipment includes ambulation aids, personal care aids, beds, therapy equipment, enteral products (e.g., pumps, tubes), and wound care equipment. Disposable supplies are those used to attend to wounds and skin, such as bandages, ostomy supplies, and syringes. Pharmaceuticals are medications and the information and materials necessary to facilitate compliance and proper usage.

45. D: Warranties and manufacturers' data are included. The durable medical equipment provider is responsible for warranties and manufacturers' data for any equipment provided. However, all other criteria noted are very important to ensure that the patient or caregiver can properly use the equipment provided to achieve the identified ends. This includes avoiding any unnecessary equipment failures and rehospitalizations.

46. C: Utilization review is retrospective, while utilization management is oriented toward the present and future. Utilization review uses the three components of preauthorization, and concurrent and retrospective review to confirm that a patient's "five rights" are secured: the right service, at the right time, by the right provider, in the right place, and at the right cost. By contrast, utilization management also probes into the future by evaluating how to manage all health care needs and resources efficiently and effectively, both currently and over time.

47. B: File a grievance with the appropriate oversight agency. An insurer is required to provide timely information about the coverage of any policy they issue. Failure to do so is grounds for filing a grievance. A typical oversight entity is the state insurance commissioner, although other options may exist. When an insurer fails to respond, it may be reasonable to take alternate steps (e.g., telephone contact, contact with upper level management, certified-mail requests), but the grievance process may well be required, particularly if issues of health require a timely response.

48. A: Contact the local Medicaid field office for consultation. Medicaid field offices often maintain available provider lists. Most states prohibit health care providers from accepting any additional payments from Medicaid patients beyond the state reimbursement rate. The licensing board cannot compel a physician to accept Medicaid. Finally, Medicaid is a means-tested coverage, and recipients would be unable to afford other insurance options.

49. C: Preauthorization, concurrent, and retrospective review. Preauthorization is the preliminary review to determine and justify need and coverage eligibility. Concurrent review refers to the process of justifying the need, level of care, and quality of ongoing services. Retrospective reviews are conducted for purposes of continuous quality improvement and to ensure that services rendered and billed match the patient's coverage and eligibility criteria.

50. D: Physician. The only person who is authorized to deny services is a physician. When a decision is appealed, the claim must be reviewed by a physician who is a specialist in the service area, and the person must not be the same specialist who rendered the first denial decision. In situations where a decision is urgently needed, an "expedited appeal" can be submitted for more rapid consideration and a timely response. In some states, both a patient and the treating physician can request a "fair hearing" to address their needs and concerns on appeal.

51. B: Government insurance plan. TRICARE is the managed health care system provided by the U.S. Military Health Service System. There are three levels of TRICARE: Prime, Standard, and Extra. All members of the military on active duty are automatically enrolled in Prime. Other forms of government insurance include: Medicare (for the elderly and certain disabled persons: Parts: A (hospital), B (outpatient and physician), C ("Plus Choice" by private point-of-service providers), and D (prescription drug coverage); Medicaid (insurance for the low-income or disabled); State Children's Health Insurance Program; and Department of Veterans Affairs insurance (coverage for military veterans).

52. A: Private health insurance plans. HMO refers to a "health maintenance organization," which provides predetermined benefits in a specific geographic location for a set periodic price. PPO refers to a "preferred provider organization" in which contracts with specific health care providers are created, thereby resulting in lower costs to the insurer and member and a consistent supply of patients for the providers. POS refers to a "point-of-service" plan that may offer both HMO and PPO options, at varying charges and rates for optimum member flexibility.

53. C: Medical expenses reimbursement of an insurer or self-insured employer out of a third-part settlement. There are times when patient's medical expenses are met by a primary insurer, but where the illness or injury is a consequence of an event or

circumstances that is otherwise covered elsewhere. For example, an on-the-job injury may be treated through the patient's primary insurer but is actually covered by Workman's Compensation, or injuries sustained in an automobile accident may later be covered under a lawsuit settlement. In such situations the insurer or a self-insured employer may be entitled to repayment by means of subrogation.

54. D: Predetermined rates for diagnostic-related groups. The 1983 Prospective Pay System created 492 diagnostic-related groups and revised Medicare reimbursement from variable fee-for-service system to a fixed price formula for services rendered. The system required hospitals to focus on four key issues: (1) reducing resource costs; (2) limiting length of stay; (3) service intensity reductions; and (4) greater efficiency in service delivery.

55. B: Comparison of products, services, and practices among different providers or leaders in a given specialty. The production of product, service, and specialty-specific benchmarks supplies ongoing performance data for subsequent comparisons. High-quality performance achievements become the benchmarks for regional and national standards, against which all others are measured. Continuous measurement and reporting allow for ongoing improvements and mutual learning.

56. A: Centers for Medicare and Medicaid Services. The Quality Improvement Organization's endeavor is to ensure "the right care for every person every time." The Joint Commission is a private organization that evaluates and accredits 15,000 health organizations and programs. The National Quality Forum is a national nonprofit organization funded by the Robert Wood Johnson Foundation and is dedicated to quality improvement in health care. The National Committee for Quality Assurance seeks to improve health care quality. Another accrediting body is the "Utilization Review Accreditation Commission," sometimes also identified as the "American Accreditation HealthCare Commission," which provides standardized utilization review criteria and certification or accreditation for more than a dozen systems and programs.

57. C: A neutral source of assistance to address the health care service concerns of local citizens. Ombudsmen are public employees who operate through an ombudsman program to provide confidential, independent assistance in addressing health services, problems, and conflicts when other options have failed. Originally established as a "Long Term Care Ombudsman" demonstration project in 1972, the program was expanded nationally in 1974 via the federal Administration on Aging. There are now more than 2,400 ombudsman programs nationwide. They assist individuals in a variety of residential care settings with, for example, quality of care, resident rights, financial concerns, allegations of abuse, and witnessing of advance directives.

58. C: Comparison of relevant benchmark data to determine services, processes, or functions that produce superior outcomes. By means of comparative benchmark analyses, providers or organizations are able to set optimized standards for the services, processes, and functions necessary to achieve enhanced clinical outcomes, increased efficiency, and lower costs. Peer review is often an essential component in establishing and maintaining the changes identified as necessary through the benchmarking and best practices profiling process.

59. D: Varying the techniques used for optimum results. Variation in the techniques applied can confound the learning and revision process, as it may not then be clear what has ultimately helped or hindered the outcome. As promoted by the Agency for Health Care Policy and Research, evidence-based practice involves: (1) identification of a problem, (2) completion of a literature and resource review, (3) the critical evaluation of available evidence for validity, (4) the application of optimal evidence, and (5) the evaluation of outcomes and revision of the intervention as needed.

60. D: All of the above. Sources of variance in care management plans and clinical pathways arise in many different ways, depending on the pathway, the patient, the diagnosis, the system resources, and other secondary influences. Consequently, "variance tracking" is extremely important. Variance tracking is initiated whenever a patient fails to progress as expected or when identified steps in a clinical pathway are missed or are left incomplete. All variances must be documented and examined, both individually and collectively, to identify all elements of influence. In certain circumstances, the clinical pathway may need to be modified to accommodate unique patient or situational factors.

61. D: Approval of the goal from accreditation or credentialing programs. Some goals may be imposed by accreditation or credentialing programs, as a condition for certification or formal accreditation after a site review. However, many more goals or quality improvement aims must arise internally, if programs and facilities are to function well and are to achieve their stated missions successfully. Thus, continuous quality improvement is an endless journey toward improvement that must be reassessed, reevaluated, and further pursued for program excellence to be maintained.

62. B: Plan, do, study, and act. The current "plan, do, study, and act" (PDSA) model is based on Shewhart's agricultural model of 1939 (specifications, production, inspection). It was refined from PDCA (plan, do, check, and act) into the PDSA cycle in 1986 and promoted by quality improvement educator William Edwards Deming. The "plan" phase refers to problem clarification and information gathering. The "do" phase is an experimental stage. The "study" phase refers to formal analysis of the results of the interventions as carried out. Finally, the "act" phase refers to formal adoption of the improvements realized.

63. C: Six sigma model. The "six sigma" model is a data-driven approach that refers to the performance of a process within six standard deviations of the mean and the closest specification limit (but not to exceed more than 3.4 defects per million instances). The "define, measure, analyze, improve, and control" model addresses incremental improvement needs, while the "define, measure, analyze, design, and verify" model is used for new products or processes or those requiring more than incremental changes. The Shewhart cycle refers to the "plan, do, check, and act" cycle, while the Deming cycle refers to the "plan, do, study, and act" cycle. Continuous quality improvement is an umbrella term encompassing all quality-improvement activities.

64. B: Specific Centers for Medicare and Medicaid Services–required quality-control measures. The Centers for Medicare and Medicaid Services mandate that health care facilities receive Medicare funds to meet certain quality standards in specified "core measures." The overall core measures are: access to services, antidiscrimination, confidentiality, and quality assurance. For hospitals, the clinical quality assurance core

measures must include protocols covering acute myocardial infarction, heart failure, pneumonia, pregnancy and related conditions, and surgical infection prevention.

65. D: Provide standardized health care quality measures. The National Quality Forum (NQF) is a nonprofit public–private partnership that was established in 1999 in response to a presidential commission. It standardizes quality performance measures and practices used in the delivery of health care. More than 400 standardized measures and practices have been endorsed, with more being added regularly. There are currently 15 NQF-endorsed consensus standards in the Nursing Care Performance Measures project, including both measures of processes and outcomes. The overarching goal is to ensure the maintenance of high-quality health care in the United States.

66. A: Problem prevention versus problem analysis and liability control. Quality management attempts to put programs, policies, and practices into play that will prevent the occurrence of health care problems. Risk management is focused on analyzing problems that have already occurred. Risk managers respond to reports of unusual occurrences and target particularly high-risk areas (e.g., medication errors, falls). Four key risk assessment steps include: (1) clarifying the level of the health hazard; (2) evaluating potential adverse health effects; (3) determining the likelihood and level of an occurrence; and (4) constructing a "dose-response model," reflecting the concentration or intensity at which illness or death may occur. Then a "risk characterization" model can be derived, revealing populations and situations at greatest risk.

67. A: Negotiation. Empathy allows the nurse case manager to take the perspective of the patient and to understand resistance. Clear and honest communication aids in nurturing trust and commitment, as well as in assessing the patient's readiness to undertake a change. Because patients are typically resistant to change, it is essential that the case manager have ethical boundaries in managing their resistance. Often the case manager must not only motivate but also challenge and confront the patient during the process of change; it is essential that the safeguards to negotiation remain in place. In this way, the patient retains autonomy and dignity even as the case manager supplies the motivation necessary to induce change.

68. C: Self-determination. Individuals have the right to make their own decisions, and others must respect their unique values, goals, and personal independence. The right to autonomy persists even if the outcomes or consequences are perceived by others to be negative. While patients must be properly informed about untoward outcomes and consequences, the competent and informed patient has the right to make choices that may be problematic. Helping the patient to explore all choices, however, is essential. Four additional guiding ethical principles include "beneficence" (the obligation to try and promote good), nonmalfeasance (the requirement to avoid doing harm), justice (the principle of fairness), and veracity (the obligation to be truthful).

69. D: Authorized access versus the right to self-disclose. Confidentiality specifically refers to the protection of externally held information, regarding an individual or group, from all but those explicitly authorized to that information. Privacy refers to the right of an individual or group to reveal or disclose itself or information about itself on a selective basis. Both are individual rights with certain limits. For example, information about certain communicable diseases may require reporting under law to protect others. However,

patient information should generally be released only to the extent required and only to the degree that it will benefit the patient and protect others.

70. B: Protect private health information. The Health Insurance Portability and Accountability (HIPPA) Act of 1996 limits the release of private health care information without the written (usually) consent of the individual. The regulation does not apply to information needed for treatment, billing, some emergency care, business planning activities, peer review, quality assurance, staff education, and research authorized by the Institutional Review Board. The "privacy rule" applies to "individually identifiable information," which is referred to as "Protected Health Information." The Health and Human Services Office for Civil Rights is responsible for implementation and enforcement of the HIPPA Act.

71. D: Deletion or removal of negative personal health information from a treating provider's records. The health provider has the right, and indeed an obligation, to maintain accurate health records regarding all patients being treated. Even if a patient has a history of treatment for an awkward or sensitive health issue, the patient does not have the right to demand that the information be removed from his or her health records. The patient does, however, have a right to confidentiality and privacy and the assurance that the health information is properly protected.

72. A: Decisional capacity is lost. Decisional capacity is the term for incompetence outside a courtroom; for example, only a judge can decree incompetence, while a properly trained clinician can certify a loss of decisional capacity. Many "statutory" advance directives speak only to limited conditions, such as terminal illness, permanent coma (unconsciousness), and a "persistent vegetative state," leading some to believe that "living wills" cannot address other issues. However, the U.S. Supreme Court has repeatedly confirmed the right of an individual to consent to or refuse any and all forms of medical treatment via a "living will" in any health care condition, provided the individual possessed decisional capacity when the choice was made (see: Cruzan, 497 U.S. 261 (1990) and the Schiavo Docket No. 04A-825).

73. C: Intentional torts. Conduct that constitutes an "intentional tort" is a planned act. The outcome may not have been intended, but the act was considered and then carried out intentionally.

74. D: Quasi-intentional torts. A quasi-intentional tort is an act that results in damage to the dignity or economics of an individual.

75. A: Unintentional torts. An unintentional tort is an act that harms unintentionally, resulting from a failure to provide a proper professional response. The "reasonable and prudent" standard refers to the application of "average" judgment and skill as expected within the profession. Consequently, it is possible to be charged with both negligence and malpractice concurrently. Four elements are required: (1) there was a duty to act; (2) the duty was breached; (3) the failure was the cause of the harm, and (4) harm or damage resulted.

76. C: The willful failure to be responsible for a person for whom one has a caregiving duty. The basis of the duty may be assignment by employment, assignment as a volunteer, or simply holding oneself as a caregiver by performing the role to the extent that others would

reasonably expect that continued care will be provided. Thus, abandonment is not setting-specific, and it can occur as readily in a home as in a formal facility. Signs of abandonment include extended caregiver absences and signs of physical neglect (e.g., bedsores, emaciation). The level of legal response depends on whether the abandonment was intentional or unintentional and on the laws of the specific state involved. Abandonment of an older dependent adult typically falls under elder abuse laws, and in some states, it may trigger a mandated report.

77. B: Low-to-moderate stress. In the total absence of stress, learning tends to be lackadaisical and unproductive. In situations of moderate-to-high stress, learning is somewhat blunted, and in high-stress circumstances, learning is significantly impaired. Consequently, the design of an educational program should challenge but not overwhelm the learners. One way to gauge the effectiveness of a learning experience is by asking the participants how they feel (i.e., relaxed, motivated, overwhelmed), which can inform the educator how well the presentation pace suits the learners.

78. C: Use both positive and negative reinforcement strategies. Reinforcement is essential to motivate change, encourage the adoption of correct behavior, and discourage incorrect behavior. Positive reinforcement is primarily used to motivate the assimilation of needed positive behaviors and changes. Negative reinforcement is principally used to dissuade and extinguish negative behaviors that must be overcome. By the consistent use of reinforcement, the case manager can aid patients in adopting needed behaviors and assist in diminishing negative behaviors, which may ultimately disappear.

79. D: Amount of practice incorporated into the learning experience. While there are many elements that can influence information retention, the most crucial element is the amount of practice that is incorporated into the learning experience. Other factors include the use of language that is easily understood, demonstrating how the information is personally relevant and applicable, and making the learning experience enjoyable by selecting an engaging style of delivery.

80. A: Self-direction, learning readiness, and a problem-centered orientation to learning. Adult learners are more likely to adopt positive health practices when they believe they are at risk of developing a specific condition, when the practices or behaviors will reduce the specific risks, when the condition involved is perceived as serious and burdened with negative consequences, and when they perceive that relevant barriers can be overcome.

81. B: Perceptual modality, information processing, and personality patterns. The perceptual modality refers to sensorial-based learning (i.e., auditory, visual, olfactory, kinesthetic), which should influence the form of presentation used for optimal learning experiences. The information processing style refers to the preferred manner of receiving, organizing, and retaining information, which also shapes processes of recall and problem-solving. Finally, the personality pattern of learning emphasizes attention, emotion, and values, all of which influence the way individuals respond to situations and circumstantial demands.

82. C: Culture and language. Culture and language are often a substantial determinant of behaviors that directly affect health and wellness. Both of these elements also substantially shape health expectations and attitudes toward health care and medical providers. Cultural

and language incompatibility often produces barriers to health care interactions and may at times be key determinants in the success or failure of proposed treatments and interventions. Mutual respect, cultural insights, and the use of interpreters where language barriers exist are all important ways to overcome the barriers that may arise.

83. D: Literacy. One of the greatest barriers to quality health care is that of poor health literacy, as some 90 million Americans have difficulty understanding and following the health information provided to them. At particular risk are the aged (half of all Medicare recipients read below the fifth grade level), immigrant populations, the economically disadvantaged, and individuals with chronic physical or mental health conditions. These groups have particular difficulties reading and comprehending health brochures, procedure-related instructions, and prescription medicine labels. This underscores the need to design basic and effective literature that meets the needs of all recipients.

84. A: An interpreter works with spoken language, and a translator deals with written language. The use of a professional interpreter with patients who have "limited English proficiency" is particularly important. While medical staff often may use relatives, friends, or nonmedical facility employees, this can be problematic. Issues of confidentiality, open expression, and proper understanding of medical terms, for example, make the need for professional interpreters and translators clear.

85. D: Assess, diagnose, identify outcomes, plan, implement, and evaluate. The text, "Nursing: Scope and Standards of Practice" thoroughly addresses the practice of nursing. It includes the "Six Standards of Practice," the "Nine Standards of Professional Performance," the seven elements of the "Bill of Rights for Registered Nurses," and the nine principles embodied in the "Code of Ethics for Nurses." It also covers practice standards for twenty-one nursing specialties, such as gerontology, psychiatry, and neonatal nursing.

86. B: Measurement guidelines. The Case Management Society of America has provided specific "measurement guidelines" to assist case managers to use effectively the standards of practice that have been provided. Each guideline offers clarification regarding the scope and application of the corresponding practice standard. Thus, for example, the case management practice standard of "planning" articulates the need for the case manager to gather relevant information comprehensively by interviews, research, and data collection sufficient to produce a clinical basis for the formulation of an appropriate plan of care.

87. C: Licensure is a legal form of professional validation, while certification refers to competence in a specialized area of a profession. A license is typically issued by a state governmental body, while certification is more frequently issued by a professional oversight organization. Both licensure and certification involve evidence of appropriate educational attainment, as well as passing further exams to ensure competency in the area of relevant practice. By contrast, possession of a "certificate" normally indicates attendance or participation in a program, activity, or meeting but does not involve testing or competency evaluation.

88. B: Milliman addresses treatment guidelines, while InterQual addresses continuum of care. Milliman care guidelines were not established to constrain treatment options but rather to offer guidelines and establish a baseline for what is possible in various care settings. The guidelines incorporate patient education tools and measures of quality

outcomes. InterQual clinical decision support tools can assist in determining an optimal path and timing of progression through the continuum of care. The goal is to derive high-quality care at the most appropriate cost and with the optimum outcome.

89. C: Descriptive, evaluative, and predictive. Descriptive screening tools collect data about population characteristics, often to identify areas of greatest need. Evaluative screening tools attempt to measure the effectiveness of health interventions and processes, such as disease management education. Predictive tools attempt to infer particular outcomes in a population as derived from lifestyle factors and disease conditions.

90. D: Short-form 36 health survey. The short-form 36 health survey (SF-36) is composed of 36 questions about health and well-being. It does not target any specific disease but functions as a generic measure of overall wellness. It can be reduced to eight profiles of functional health and well-being. The eight scales can also be configured to form two physical and mental health clusters. The SF-36 has a proven record of reliability and validity and has been useful in general and specific populations and in comparing the relative burdens associated with various disease processes. It has also been used to evaluate the health benefits of varying treatment interventions.

91. A: Clinical practice guidelines. Clinical practice guidelines (or simply clinical guidelines) are designed to guide practitioners, ancillary health care providers, patients, and family caregivers to determine appropriate health care options in carefully defined circumstances. The guidelines are derived from research and practice outcomes and attempt to provide optimum care with limited resources. There is normally a significant time lapse from the introduction of clinical practice guidelines to full adoption in the practical setting, typically about 17 years.

92. C: Clinical pathway. Also known as a "clinical care practice," a "clinical care map," or a "best practices pathway," these structured, multidisciplinary plans of care are designed to aid in the process of optimum clinical and resource management. They are arranged in a stepwise sequence and typically have four key components: (1) a timeline, (2) categories of care or needed interventions, (3) expected outcome criteria, and (4) prompts for variance tracking. Algorithms, guidelines, and protocols differ from a pathway in that it is used by a multidisciplinary team and emphasizes care coordination and quality.

93. D: They both use stepwise sequencing, but algorithms are supported by research-based data. Perhaps the best known algorithm is that used in rendering advanced cardiac life support. The algorithm is guided by the kind of cardiac rhythm in evidence, which prompts specific clinical responses on the part of medical practitioners during a resuscitation effort. Algorithms are particularly helpful in emergency situations, and in situations where the medical options are diverse and complex.

94. A: A situation that does not clearly present a best course of action. This often occurs when only limited or incomplete information is available, and circumstances require timely intervention. At such times, it may be necessary to estimate the optimum course of treatment or intervention. In certain circumstances, decision trees may also be computerized to aid in analyzing the relevant information and determining a most likely course of action. The goal is to optimize outcomes, reduce treatment variation, and improve guideline compliance.

95. B: Centers for Medicare and Medicaid Services. Multiple agencies have been involved in designing the Consumer Assessment of Healthcare Provider and Systems (CAHPS) surveys as unique CAHPS surveys needed to be designed for a variety of settings, such as hospitals, dialysis centers, and nursing homes. Consequently, a consortium of entities, such as the Agency for Healthcare Research and Quality, National Committee for Quality Assurance, and others, collaborated in designing these surveys. However, they are administered under the auspices of the Centers for Medicare and Medicaid Services.

96. B: 1990. The informal roots of case management extend back into the early 1980s, and a leadership meeting in Chicago later that decade led to the establishment of the Case Management Society of America (CMSA) in 1990. The first certification exam was held in 1993, sponsored by the Commission for Case Management Certification. In 1995, the CMSA was the first organization to produce "Standards of Practice." While case management is a multidisciplinary field of practice, the majority of case managers are nurses.

97. A: Preceptorship is formal and supervisory, while mentoring is informal and is less instructional. Preceptors pursue an organized tutorial relationship, provide technical assistance, and offer direct supervision during a discrete period of time. Mentors focus on professional growth through consultation and advising. A substantive component is the use of role modeling and practicum in the development of a skilled case manager.

98. D: Staff development. Continuing education refers to outside programs that offer instructional programs needed to maintain licensure. Other similar opportunities include conferences and professional training courses of instruction. Whenever educational opportunities are sponsored by an organization for its employees, release time is provided, or an educational opportunity is broadcast and encouraged, it falls under the term "staff development." It is important for organizations to maintain records of staff development programs and attendance, as they may be part of an accreditation review at some future time.

99. C: Performance appraisals, peer review, and self-evaluation. While meetings, surveys, discussions, and collaborations may offer insight into the performance of employees or contractees, the "essential" tools for evaluation are very direct and specific. All staff and contractees should engage in continuing education and professional development, but management must also engage in the direct and ongoing assessment and evaluation of employee/contractee competencies. Any independently practicing professional should conduct regular self-assessments and engage in continuing education to ensure quality skills and professional competency.

100. C: Professional who holds a license, certification, or credential. Although many other parties, including patients and other consumers of health care, hold a vested interest in professionals having appropriate skills and competencies, the primary burden of remaining current and up-to-date in one's profession rests squarely on the professional. He or she should attend conferences, maintain membership in professional organizations, read professional journals, participate in continuing education and research, and attempt to keep current in the profession in any way possible.

Special Report: What Your Test Score Will Tell You About Your IQ

Did you know that most standardized tests correlate very strongly with IQ? In fact, your general intelligence is a better predictor of your success than any other factor, and most tests intentionally measure this trait to some degree to ensure that those selected by the test are truly qualified for the test's purposes.

Before we can delve into the relation between your test score and IQ, I will first have to explain what exactly is IQ. Here's the formula:

Your IQ = 100 + (Number of standard deviations below or above the average)*15

Now, let's define standard deviations by using an example. If we have 5 people with 5 different heights, then first we calculate the average. Let's say the average was 65 inches. The standard deviation is the "average distance" away from the average of each of the members. It is a direct measure of variability - if the 5 people included Jackie Chan and Shaquille O'Neal, obviously there's a lot more variability in that group than a group of 5 sisters who are all within 6 inches in height of each other. The standard deviation uses a number to characterize the average range of difference within a group.

A convenient feature of most groups is that they have a "normal" distribution- makes sense that most things would be normal, right? Without getting into a bunch of statistical mumbo-jumbo, you just need to know that if you know the average of the group and the standard deviation, you can successfully predict someone's percentile rank in the group.

Confused? Let me give you an example. If instead of 5 people's heights, we had 100 people, we could figure out their rank in height JUST by knowing the average, standard deviation, and their height. We wouldn't need to know each person's height and manually rank them; we could just predict their rank based on three numbers.

What this means is that you can take your PERCENTILE rank that is often given with your test and relate this to your RELATIVE IQ of people taking the test - that is, your IQ relative to the people taking the test. Obviously, there's no way to know your actual IQ because the people taking a standardized test are usually not very good samples of the general population- many of those with extremely low IQ's never achieve a level of success or competency necessary to complete a typical standardized test. In fact, professional psychologists who measure IQ actually have to use non-written tests that can fairly measure the IQ of those not able to complete a traditional test.

The bottom line is to not take your test score too seriously, but it is fun to compute your "relative IQ" among the people who took the test with you. I've done the calculations below. Just look up your percentile rank in the left and then you'll see your "relative IQ" for your test in the right hand column.

Percentile Rank	Your Relative IQ		Percentile Rank	Your Relative IQ
99	135		59	103
98	131		58	103
97	128		57	103
96	126		56	102
95	125		55	102
94	123		54	102
93	122		53	101
92	121		52	101
91	120		51	100
90	119		50	100
89	118		49	100
88	118		48	99
87	117		47	99
86	116		46	98
85	116		45	98
84	115		44	98
83	114		43	97
82	114		42	97
81	113		41	97
80	113		40	96
79	112		39	96
78	112		38	95
77	111		37	95
76	111		36	95
75	110		35	94
74	110		34	94
73	109		33	93
72	109		32	93
71	108		31	93
70	108		30	92
69	107		29	92
68	107		28	91
67	107		27	91
66	106		26	90
65	106		25	90
64	105		24	89
63	105		23	89
62	105		22	88
61	104		21	88
60	104		20	87

Special Report: What is Test Anxiety and How to Overcome It?

The very nature of tests caters to some level of anxiety, nervousness or tension, just as we feel for any important event that occurs in our lives. A little bit of anxiety or nervousness can be a good thing. It helps us with motivation, and makes achievement just that much sweeter. However, too much anxiety can be a problem; especially if it hinders our ability to function and perform.

"Test anxiety," is the term that refers to the emotional reactions that some test-takers experience when faced with a test or exam. Having a fear of testing and exams is based upon a rational fear, since the test-taker's performance can shape the course of an academic career. Nevertheless, experiencing excessive fear of examinations will only interfere with the test-takers ability to perform and his/her chances to be successful.

There are a large variety of causes that can contribute to the development and sensation of test anxiety. These include, but are not limited to lack of performance and worrying about issues surrounding the test.

Lack of Preparation

Lack of preparation can be identified by the following behaviors or situations:

Not scheduling enough time to study, and therefore cramming the night before the test or exam
Managing time poorly, to create the sensation that there is not enough time to do everything
Failing to organize the text information in advance, so that the study material consists of the entire text and not simply the pertinent information
Poor overall studying habits

Worrying, on the other hand, can be related to both the test taker, and many other factors around him/her that will be affected by the results of the test. These include worrying about:

Previous performances on similar exams, or exams in general
How friends and other students are achieving
The negative consequences that will result from a poor grade or failure

There are three primary elements to test anxiety. Physical components which involve the same typical bodily reactions as those to acute anxiety (to be discussed below).

Emotional factors have to do with fear or panic. Mental or cognitive issues concerning attention spans and memory abilities.

Physical Signals

There are many different symptoms of test anxiety, and these are not limited to mental and emotional strain. Frequently there are a range of physical signals that will let a test taker know that he/she is suffering from test anxiety. These bodily changes can include the following:

Perspiring
Sweaty palms
Wet, trembling hands
Nausea
Dry mouth
A knot in the stomach
Headache
Faintness
Muscle tension
Aching shoulders, back and neck
Rapid heart beat
Feeling too hot/cold

To recognize the sensation of test anxiety, a test-taker should monitor him/herself for the following sensations:

The physical distress symptoms as listed above
Emotional sensitivity, expressing emotional feelings such as the need to cry or laugh too much, or a sensation of anger or helplessness
A decreased ability to think, causing the test-taker to blank out or have racing thoughts that are hard to organize or control.

Though most students will feel some level of anxiety when faced with a test or exam, the majority can cope with that anxiety and maintain it at a manageable level. However, those who cannot are faced with a very real and very serious condition, which can and should be controlled for the immeasurable benefit of this sufferer.

Naturally, these sensations lead to negative results for the testing experience. The most common effects of test anxiety have to do with nervousness and mental blocking.

Nervousness

Nervousness can appear in several different levels:

The test-taker's difficulty, or even inability to read and understand the questions on the test
The difficulty or inability to organize thoughts to a coherent form
The difficulty or inability to recall key words and concepts relating to the testing questions (especially essays)
The receipt of poor grades on a test, though the test material was well known by the test taker

Conversely, a person may also experience mental blocking, which involves:

Blanking out on test questions
Only remembering the correct answers to the questions when the test has already finished.

Fortunately for test anxiety sufferers, beating these feelings, to a large degree, has to do with proper preparation. When a test taker has a feeling of preparedness, then anxiety will be dramatically lessened.

The first step to resolving anxiety issues is to distinguish which of the two types of anxiety are being suffered. If the anxiety is a direct result of a lack of preparation, this should be considered a normal reaction, and the anxiety level (as opposed to the test results) shouldn't be anything to worry about. However, if, when adequately prepared, the test-taker still panics, blanks out, or seems to overreact, this is not a fully rational reaction. While this can be considered normal too, there are many ways to combat and overcome these effects.

Remember that anxiety cannot be entirely eliminated, however, there are ways to minimize it, to make the anxiety easier to manage. Preparation is one of the best ways to minimize test anxiety. Therefore the following techniques are wise in order to best fight off any anxiety that may want to build.

To begin with, try to avoid cramming before a test, whenever it is possible. By trying to memorize an entire term's worth of information in one day, you'll be shocking your system, and not giving yourself a very good chance to absorb the information. This is an easy path to anxiety, so for those who suffer from test anxiety, cramming should not even be considered an option.

Instead of cramming, work throughout the semester to combine all of the material which is presented throughout the semester, and work on it gradually as the course goes by, making sure to master the main concepts first, leaving minor details for a week or so before the test.

To study for the upcoming exam, be sure to pose questions that may be on the examination, to gauge the ability to answer them by integrating the ideas from your texts, notes and lectures, as well as any supplementary readings.

If it is truly impossible to cover all of the information that was covered in that particular term, concentrate on the most important portions that can be covered very well. Learn these concepts as best as possible, so that when the test comes, a goal can be made to use these concepts as presentations of your knowledge.

In addition to study habits, changes in attitude are critical to beating a struggle with test anxiety. In fact, an improvement of the perspective over the entire test-taking experience can actually help a test taker to enjoy studying and therefore improve the overall experience. Be certain not to overemphasize the significance of the grade - know that the result of the test is neither a reflection of self worth, nor is it a measure of intelligence; one grade will not predict a person's future success.

To improve an overall testing outlook, the following steps should be tried:

Keeping in mind that the most reasonable expectation for taking a test is to expect to try to demonstrate as much of what you know as you possibly can.
Reminding ourselves that a test is only one test; this is not the only one, and there will be others.
The thought of thinking of oneself in an irrational, all-or-nothing term should be avoided at all costs.
A reward should be designated for after the test, so there's something to look forward to. Whether it is going to a movie, going out to eat, or simply visiting friends, schedule it in advance, and do it no matter what result is expected on the exam.

Test-takers should also keep in mind that the basics are some of the most important things, even beyond anti-anxiety techniques and studying. Never neglect the basic social, emotional and biological needs, in order to try to absorb information. In order to best achieve, these three factors must be held as just as important as the studying itself.

Study Steps

Remember the following important steps for studying:

Maintain healthy nutrition and exercise habits. Continue both your recreational activities and social pass times. These both contribute to your physical and emotional well being.
Be certain to get a good amount of sleep, especially the night before the test, because when you're overtired you are not able to perform to the best of your best ability.
Keep the studying pace to a moderate level by taking breaks when they are needed, and varying the work whenever possible, to keep the mind fresh instead of getting bored.

When enough studying has been done that all the material that can be learned has been learned, and the test taker is prepared for the test, stop studying and do something relaxing such as listening to music, watching a movie, or taking a warm bubble bath.

There are also many other techniques to minimize the uneasiness or apprehension that is experienced along with test anxiety before, during, or even after the examination. In fact, there are a great deal of things that can be done to stop anxiety from interfering with lifestyle and performance. Again, remember that anxiety will not be eliminated entirely, and it shouldn't be. Otherwise that "up" feeling for exams would not exist, and most of us depend on that sensation to perform better than usual. However, this anxiety has to be at a level that is manageable.

Of course, as we have just discussed, being prepared for the exam is half the battle right away. Attending all classes, finding out what knowledge will be expected on the exam, and knowing the exam schedules are easy steps to lowering anxiety. Keeping up with work will remove the need to cram, and efficient study habits will eliminate wasted time. Studying should be done in an ideal location for concentration, so that it is simple to become interested in the material and give it complete attention. A method such as SQ3R (Survey, Question, Read, Recite, Review) is a wonderful key to follow to make sure that the study habits are as effective as possible, especially in the case of learning from a textbook. Flashcards are great techniques for memorization. Learning to take good notes will mean that notes will be full of useful information, so that less sifting will need to be done to seek out what is pertinent for studying. Reviewing notes after class and then again on occasion will keep the information fresh in the mind. From notes that have been taken summary sheets and outlines can be made for simpler reviewing.

A study group can also be a very motivational and helpful place to study, as there will be a sharing of ideas, all of the minds can work together, to make sure that everyone understands, and the studying will be made more interesting because it will be a social occasion.

Basically, though, as long as the test-taker remains organized and self confident, with efficient study habits, less time will need to be spent studying, and higher grades will be achieved.

To become self confident, there are many useful steps. The first of these is "self talk." It has been shown through extensive research, that self-talk for students who suffer from test anxiety, should be well monitored, in order to make sure that it contributes to self confidence as opposed to sinking the student. Frequently the self talk of test-anxious students is negative or self-defeating, thinking that everyone else is smarter and faster, that they always mess up, and that if they don't do well, they'll fail the entire course. It is important to decreasing anxiety that awareness is made of self talk. Try writing any negative self thoughts and then disputing them with a positive statement instead. Begin self-encouragement as though it was a friend speaking. Repeat positive statements to help reprogram the mind to believing in successes instead of failures.

Helpful Techniques

Other extremely helpful techniques include:

Self-visualization of doing well and reaching goals
While aiming for an "A" level of understanding, don't try to "overprotect" by setting your expectations lower. This will only convince the mind to stop studying in order to meet the lower expectations.
Don't make comparisons with the results or habits of other students. These are individual factors, and different things work for different people, causing different results.
Strive to become an expert in learning what works well, and what can be done in order to improve. Consider collecting this data in a journal.
Create rewards for after studying instead of doing things before studying that will only turn into avoidance behaviors.
Make a practice of relaxing - by using methods such as progressive relaxation, self-hypnosis, guided imagery, etc - in order to make relaxation an automatic sensation.
Work on creating a state of relaxed concentration so that concentrating will take on the focus of the mind, so that none will be wasted on worrying.
Take good care of the physical self by eating well and getting enough sleep.
Plan in time for exercise and stick to this plan.

Beyond these techniques, there are other methods to be used before, during and after the test that will help the test-taker perform well in addition to overcoming anxiety.

Before the exam comes the academic preparation. This involves establishing a study schedule and beginning at least one week before the actual date of the test. By doing this, the anxiety of not having enough time to study for the test will be automatically eliminated. Moreover, this will make the studying a much more effective experience, ensuring that the learning will be an easier process. This relieves much undue pressure on the test-taker.

Summary sheets, note cards, and flash cards with the main concepts and examples of these main concepts should be prepared in advance of the actual studying time. A topic should never be eliminated from this process. By omitting a topic because it isn't expected to be on the test is only setting up the test-taker for anxiety should it actually appear on the exam. Utilize the course syllabus for laying out the topics that should be studied. Carefully go over the notes that were made in class, paying special attention to any of the issues that the professor took special care to emphasize while lecturing in class. In the textbooks, use the chapter review, or if possible, the chapter tests, to begin your review.

It may even be possible to ask the instructor what information will be covered on the exam, or what the format of the exam will be (for example, multiple choice, essay, free form, true-false). Additionally, see if it is possible to find out how many questions will be on the test. If a review sheet or sample test has been offered by the professor, make good use of it, above anything else, for the preparation for the test. Another great resource for getting to know the examination is reviewing tests from previous semesters. Use these tests to review, and aim to achieve a 100% score on each of the possible topics. With a few exceptions, the goal that you set for yourself is the highest one that you will reach.

Take all of the questions that were assigned as homework, and rework them to any other possible course material. The more problems reworked, the more skill and confidence will form as a result. When forming the solution to a problem, write out each of the steps. Don't simply do head work. By doing as many steps on paper as possible, much clarification and therefore confidence will be formed. Do this with as many homework problems as possible, before checking the answers. By checking the answer after each problem, reinforcement will exist, that will not be on the exam. Study situations should be as exam-like as possible, to prime the test-taker's system for the experience. By waiting to check the answers at the end, a psychological advantage will be formed, to decrease the stress factor.

Another fantastic reason for not cramming is the avoidance of confusion in concepts, especially when it comes to mathematics. 8-10 hours of study will become one hundred percent more effective if it is spread out over a week or at least several days, instead of doing it all in one sitting. Recognize that the human brain requires time in order to assimilate new material, so frequent breaks and a span of study time over several days will be much more beneficial.

Additionally, don't study right up until the point of the exam. Studying should stop a minimum of one hour before the exam begins. This allows the brain to rest and put things in their proper order. This will also provide the time to become as relaxed as possible when going into the examination room. The test-taker will also have time to eat well and eat sensibly. Know that the brain needs food as much as the rest of the body. With enough food and enough sleep, as well as a relaxed attitude, the body and the mind are primed for success.

Avoid any anxious classmates who are talking about the exam. These students only spread anxiety, and are not worth sharing the anxious sentimentalities.

Before the test also involves creating a positive attitude, so mental preparation should also be a point of concentration. There are many keys to creating a positive attitude. Should fears become rushing in, make a visualization of taking the exam, doing well, and seeing an A written on the paper. Write out a list of affirmations that will bring a feeling of confidence, such as "I am doing well in my English class," "I studied well and know my material," "I enjoy this class." Even if the affirmations aren't believed at first, it sends a positive message to the subconscious which will result in an alteration of the overall belief system, which is the system that creates reality.

If a sensation of panic begins, work with the fear and imagine the very worst! Work through the entire scenario of not passing the test, failing the entire course, and dropping out of school, followed by not getting a job, and pushing a shopping cart through the dark alley where you'll live. This will place things into perspective! Then, practice deep breathing and create a visualization of the opposite situation - achieving an "A" on the exam, passing the entire course, receiving the degree at a graduation ceremony.

On the day of the test, there are many things to be done to ensure the best results, as well as the most calm outlook. The following stages are suggested in order to maximize test-taking potential:

Begin the examination day with a moderate breakfast, and avoid any coffee or beverages with caffeine if the test taker is prone to jitters. Even people who are used to managing caffeine can feel jittery or light-headed when it is taken on a test day.
Attempt to do something that is relaxing before the examination begins. As last minute cramming clouds the mastering of overall concepts, it is better to use this time to create a calming outlook.
Be certain to arrive at the test location well in advance, in order to provide time to select a location that is away from doors, windows and other distractions, as well as giving enough time to relax before the test begins.
Keep away from anxiety generating classmates who will upset the sensation of stability and relaxation that is being attempted before the exam.
Should the waiting period before the exam begins cause anxiety, create a self-distraction by reading a light magazine or something else that is relaxing and simple.

During the exam itself, read the entire exam from beginning to end, and find out how much time should be allotted to each individual problem. Once writing the exam, should more time be taken for a problem, it should be abandoned, in order to begin another problem. If there is time at the end, the unfinished problem can always be returned to and completed.

Read the instructions very carefully - twice - so that unpleasant surprises won't follow during or after the exam has ended.

When writing the exam, pretend that the situation is actually simply the completion of homework within a library, or at home. This will assist in forming a relaxed atmosphere, and will allow the brain extra focus for the complex thinking function.

Begin the exam with all of the questions with which the most confidence is felt. This will build the confidence level regarding the entire exam and will begin a quality momentum. This will also create encouragement for trying the problems where uncertainty resides.

Going with the "gut instinct" is always the way to go when solving a problem. Second guessing should be avoided at all costs. Have confidence in the ability to do well.

For essay questions, create an outline in advance that will keep the mind organized and make certain that all of the points are remembered. For multiple choice, read every answer, even if the correct one has been spotted - a better one may exist.

Continue at a pace that is reasonable and not rushed, in order to be able to work carefully. Provide enough time to go over the answers at the end, to check for small errors that can be corrected.

Should a feeling of panic begin, breathe deeply, and think of the feeling of the body releasing sand through its pores. Visualize a calm, peaceful place, and include all of the sights, sounds and sensations of this image. Continue the deep breathing, and take a few minutes to continue this with closed eyes. When all is well again, return to the test.

If a "blanking" occurs for a certain question, skip it and move on to the next question. There will be time to return to the other question later. Get everything done that can be done, first, to guarantee all the grades that can be compiled, and to build all of the confidence possible. Then return to the weaker questions to build the marks from there.

Remember, one's own reality can be created, so as long as the belief is there, success will follow. And remember: anxiety can happen later, right now, there's an exam to be written!

After the examination is complete, whether there is a feeling for a good grade or a bad grade, don't dwell on the exam, and be certain to follow through on the reward that was promised…and enjoy it! Don't dwell on any mistakes that have been made, as there is nothing that can be done at this point anyway.

Additionally, don't begin to study for the next test right away. Do something relaxing for a while, and let the mind relax and prepare itself to begin absorbing information again.

From the results of the exam - both the grade and the entire experience, be certain to learn from what has gone on. Perfect studying habits and work some more on confidence in order to make the next examination experience even better than the last one.

Learn to avoid places where openings occurred for laziness, procrastination and day dreaming.

Use the time between this exam and the next one to better learn to relax, even learning to relax on cue, so that any anxiety can be controlled during the next exam. Learn how to relax the body. Slouch in your chair if that helps. Tighten and then relax all of the different muscle groups, one group at a time, beginning with the feet and then working all the way up to the neck and face. This will ultimately relax the muscles more than they were to begin with. Learn how to breathe deeply and comfortably, and focus on this breathing going in and out as a relaxing thought. With every exhale, repeat the word "relax."

As common as test anxiety is, it is very possible to overcome it. Make yourself one of the test-takers who overcome this frustrating hindrance.

Special Report: Retaking the Test: What Are Your Chances at Improving Your Score?

After going through the experience of taking a major test, many test takers feel that once is enough. The test usually comes during a period of transition in the test taker's life, and taking the test is only one of a series of important events. With so many distractions and conflicting recommendations, it may be difficult for a test taker to rationally determine whether or not he should retake the test after viewing his scores.

The importance of the test usually only adds to the burden of the retake decision. However, don't be swayed by emotion. There a few simple questions that you can ask yourself to guide you as you try to determine whether a retake would improve your score:

1. What went wrong? Why wasn't your score what you expected?

Can you point to a single factor or problem that you feel caused the low score? Were you sick on test day? Was there an emotional upheaval in your life that caused a distraction? Were you late for the test or not able to use the full time allotment? If you can point to any of these specific, individual problems, then a retake should definitely be considered.

2. Is there enough time to improve?

Many problems that may show up in your score report may take a lot of time for improvement. A deficiency in a particular math skill may require weeks or months of tutoring and studying to improve. If you have enough time to improve an identified weakness, then a retake should definitely be considered.

3. How will additional scores be used? Will a score average, highest score, or most recent score be used?

Different test scores may be handled completely differently. If you've taken the test multiple times, sometimes your highest score is used, sometimes your average score is computed and used, and sometimes your most recent score is used. Make sure you understand what method will be used to evaluate your scores, and use that to help you determine whether a retake should be considered.

4. Are my practice test scores significantly higher than my actual test score?

If you have taken a lot of practice tests and are consistently scoring at a much higher level than your actual test score, then you should consider a retake. However, if you've taken five practice tests and only one of your scores was higher than your actual test score, or if your practice test scores were only slightly higher than your actual test score, then it is unlikely that you will significantly increase your score.

5. Do I need perfect scores or will I be able to live with this score? Will this score still allow me to follow my dreams?

What kind of score is acceptable to you? Is your current score "good enough?" Do you have to have a certain score in order to pursue the future of your dreams? If you won't be happy with your current score, and there's no way that you could live with it, then you should consider a retake. However, don't get your hopes up. If you are looking for significant improvement, that may or may not be possible. But if you won't be happy otherwise, it is at least worth the effort.
Remember that there are other considerations. To achieve your dream, it is likely that your grades may also be taken into account. A great test score is usually not the only thing necessary to succeed. Make sure that you aren't overemphasizing the importance of a high test score.

Furthermore, a retake does not always result in a higher score. Some test takers will score lower on a retake, rather than higher. One study shows that one-fourth of test takers will achieve a significant improvement in test score, while one-sixth of test takers will actually show a decrease. While this shows that most test takers will improve, the majority will only improve their scores a little and a retake may not be worth the test taker's effort.

Finally, if a test is taken only once and is considered in the added context of good grades on the part of a test taker, the person reviewing the grades and scores may be tempted to assume that the test taker just had a bad day while taking the test, and may discount the low test score in favor of the high grades. But if the test is retaken and the scores are approximately the same, then the validity of the low scores are only confirmed. Therefore, a retake could actually hurt a test taker by definitely bracketing a test taker's score ability to a limited range.

Special Report: Additional Bonus Material

Due to our efforts to try to keep this book to a manageable length, we've created a link that will give you access to all of your additional bonus material.

Please visit http://www.mometrix.com/bonus948/ccm to access the information.